Sexual Transmission of HIV Infection: Risk Reduction, Trauma, and Adaptation

Sexual Transmission of HIV Infection: Risk Reduction, Trauma and Adaptation

Lena Nilsson Schönnesson, PhD
Editor

The Haworth Press, Inc.
New York • London • Norwood (Australia)

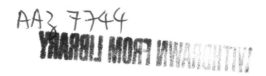

Sexual Transmission of HIV Infection: Risk Reduction, Trauma, and Adaptation has also been published as *Journal of Psychology & Human Sexuality*, Volume 5, Numbers 1/2 1992.

The Haworth Press, Inc., 10 Alice Street, Binghamton, NY 13904-1580 USA

Library of Congress Cataloging-in-Publication Data

Sexual transmission of HIV infection: risk reduction, trauma, and adaptation / Lena Nilsson Schönnesson, Editor
    p. cm.
    "Has also been published as Journal of psychology & human sexuality, volume 5, numbers 1/2 1992"-t.p. verso.
    Includes bibliographical references.
    ISBN 1-56024-332-5 (H: alk paper):-ISBN 1-56023-024-X (HPP: alk. paper)
    1. HIV infections-Transmission. 2. HIV infections-Prevention 3. HIV infections-Psychological aspects. 4. HIV infections-Risk factors. I. Schönnesson, Lena Nilsson
    [DNLM: 1. HIV Infections-prevention & control. 2. HIV infections-psychology. 3. HIV infections-transmission. 4. Risk factors. 5. Sex Behavior-psychology. W1 JO858B v.5 nos. 1/2]
RC607.A26S46 1992
616.97'9205-dc20
DNLM/DLC
for Library of Congress
                                         92-49781
                                             CIP

Sexual Transmission of HIV Infection: Risk Reduction, Trauma, and Adaptation

Sexual Transmission of HIV Infection: Risk Reduction, Trauma, and Adaptation

CONTENTS

ABOUT THE EDITOR

Lena Nilsson Schönnesson, PhD, is a licensed psychologist at the PH-Center, a psychosocial center for gay and bisexual men in Stockholm, Sweden. She also supervises health personnel at an HIV-Clinic for gay and bisexual men and lectures about HIV and sexuality. Currently, Dr. Schönnesson is completing a research report on trauma, adaptation, and psychological well-being among homosexual HIV-carriers, for which she has studied twenty-nine men for over a year. She has been a temporary advisor to the World Health Organization on issues related to human sexuality and psychosocial aspects on HIV.

Sexual Transmission of HIV Infection: Risk Reduction, Trauma, and Adaptation

Preface

I am honored and pleased to edit this volume on human immunodeficiency virus (HIV) and I am very proud of the articles presented. Different as they may seem in content, methodology, and theoretical perspective, they have a common goal: they all strive to illuminate the complexities and the dynamics of sexual risk reduction and of the existential and adaptation aspects of HIV.

It is generally agreed upon that attitudinal and behavioral changes in sex and IV drug use are the primary methods of HIV-prevention. Since men who have sex with other men have accounted for the vast majority of cases of HIV, most empirical research on sexual behavior risk reduction has so far been conducted in this population. In other words, the extent to which heterosexual and bisexual women and men, IV drug users, young people, people with different ethnic background, etc., have changed their potential risky sexual behavior is still quite unknown to us.

In order to facilitate comprehensive, effective and well-designed HIV-prevention programs it is necessary to generate knowledge as to which factors, circumstances, and conditions may obstruct/encourage sexual behavior risk reduction and its maintenance in all groups. Distressingly little attention has been paid to these central issues. Those empirical and clinical data that do exist clearly indicate that reduction in high-risk sexual behavior is not associated with information dissemination alone. There appears to be a complex relationship between factors such as information about HIV, personality, knowledge about HIV-serostatus, perceived personal susceptibility to HIV, personal efficacy about risk reduction, perceived stress and psychological cost of risk reduction, locus of control, social norms and support, beliefs about sexual enjoyability, and degree of sexual behavioral risk reduction.

In his article, Ulrich Clement addresses the underlying dynamics of unprotected intercourse among HIV-positive homosexual men.

xiii

Theo Sandfort on the other hand approaches sexual risk-taking and (mis)perception within a general Dutch population. Michael Ross's article focuses on the neglected topic of sexual behaviors in female and male heterosexual and homosexual IV drug users. In contrast to many other studies of men who have sex with men, Leif Persson and his colleagues focus on sexual contact patterns of HIV-positive homosexual men rather than on their sexual behaviors. Further, they examine the influence of psychosocial factors on sexual contact patterns.

Despite the fact that HIV infection rates among women continue to accelerate, the literature on HIV contains little discussion on women and HIV. Willeke Bezemer outlines in her article a general framework of relevant issues concerning women and HIV. HIV prevention programs specifically tailored for women are very rare. In designing effective preventive interventions, prevention strategists must acknowledge the complexities of heterosexual encounters and that the male/female negotiation of "safer sex" is shaped through the inequalities inherent in gendered power relations. Anke A. Ehrhardt and her colleagues' contribution examines the difficulties women face in ensuring protection against heterosexual HIV transmission, given these inequalities.

Although distress experienced by people with HIV transcends the medical dimensions of the disease, studies on HIV-adaptation processes, treatment or management of distress and other psychological consequences of disease progression, existential concerns on other aspects of patient care are sadly neglected in cross-sectional and longitudinal empirical research. We need more understanding of, for example, the impact of social network and support, perceived control, attributional tendencies, AIDS-induced stress, coping strategies, and coping styles on psychological wellbeing. By increasing our knowledge as to psychological processes operating within individuals who are HIV-seropositive, clinicians will be better equipped to adapt the therapeutic efforts to the patient's suffering and his/her resources and thus support and help him or her in an adequate way. Susan Schaefer and Eli Coleman's contribution and Sven-Axel Månsson's article in this volume begin to address this void, as does my own article.

I am deeply grateful to all the contributors to this volume. It is my sincere hope that the articles will be appreciated both as significant contributions to the HIV-literature and as wells of inspiration to those conducting HIV-related research or clinical work. Hopefully, too, the volume will serve as an inspiration for HIV-carriers in their fight for their right to a dignified life and a dignified death.

Lena Nilsson Schönnesson
Editor

Traumatic and Adaptation Dimensions of HIV Infection

Lena Nilsson Schönnesson, PhD

SUMMARY. The concept of "trauma" is one of the most commonly used concepts in HIV-related psychological literature. Trauma refers in this article to the intimate interplay between internal and external HIV-related threats on the one hand and emotions of helplessness, powerlessness and anxieties of separation and annihilation on the other hand. These emotional reactions can be of an existential as well as of a neurotic character. It is suggested in this article that HIV-related threats can be grouped into 3 broad areas: threats to physical existence, social existence, and sexual existence. Given these threats, HIV-carriers can suffer virtually any form of stress-related psychological and sexual dysfunctioning. To cope with, adapt to, and to learn to live with one's HIV-infection is a life-long adaptation-process. Instead of stage-crisis models, it is here argued for a model based upon the concept of adaptation. "Adaptation" refers to a subjective adaptation constituted by the individual's access to her/his psychological and social resources.

Learning that one has been infected by the HIV is a traumatic situation. "Stress" and "trauma" are the most common concepts being used in psychological literature describing HIV-related afflictions. Too often, however, the concepts are used without any real substance, thus not clarifying the strains of being an HIV-carrier. The concept of "trauma" refers in this text to the intimate interplay between internal and external HIV-related threats on the one hand and emotions of helplessness, powerlessness, and anxieties of separation and annihilation on the other hand (Weimer, Nilsson Schön-

Lena Nilsson Schönnesson is affiliated with the Ph-Center/Psychosocial Center for Gay and Bisexual Men, Box 175 31, S-118 91 Stockholm, Sweden.

1

nesson & Clement, 1990). The anxieties are basically of an existential nature, but can be reinforced and colored by neurotic anxiety. These emotional reactions can be elucidated at the time of HIV-diagnosis, but can also be activated when HIV-related symptoms/diseases start to develop, when interpersonal/sociocultural complications appear and/or intrapsychic conflicts are activated.

HIV-RELATED THREATS AND WORRIES

HIV-infection is surrounded by various worries, due to perceived threats, that can be grouped into 3 broad areas: those related to disease, dying, and death (*worries about physical existence*); others related to stigmatization and alienation (*worries about social existence*); and finally those threats and stressors related to sexual well-being (*worries about sexual existence*) (Nilsson Schönnesson, 1991).

Worries about physical existence emanate from 2 threats, one internal threat from HIV and one external threat in terms of collective representation of HIV and its prognosis. A most prominent threat to the HIV-carrier is the uncertainty in terms of disease progression, bodily deterioration and weakness, treatment, and ultimately death. Most HIV-carriers report that this uncertainty is more or less a constant on their minds, but its intensity may vary over time. These worries can be reinforced by collective representations of HIV. Mass media chooses to focus on messages of fear, of the defenseless victim of an aggressive virus, and death, rather than on the possibilities for living with the infection.

Worries about social existence originate from threats of discrimination, abandonment, and alienation as a consequence of the stigma of HIV infection. Stigmatization poses a potential risk of abandonment or alienation when disclosing one's HIV-seropositivity. Each HIV-carrier runs the risk of social expulsion.

Mass media has contributed to the stigmatization by bringing forward the invidious implications of blame and personal responsibility for one's HIV-infection. Three categories of HIV-carriers can be identified within mass media: the innocent, the suspect, and the guilty (Albert, 1986). Men who have sex with men, prostitutes, and drug users are examples of "the guilty" and are held personally responsible for their HIV-infection.

The HIV infection is thus superimposed on an already stigmatized status associated with minority group membership. The fact that HIV infection was first discerned among homosexual men has reinforced negative feelings for this group. A profound contempt for homosexuals–and self-contempt of many homosexuals–has resurfaced since apocalyptic fears have become linked with homosexuals. The impact of HIV on public attitudes toward homosexuals has lead to many instances of overt discrimination, social ostracism, deprivation of human rights and violence.

Worries about sexual existence. Frustration and stress around the need to engage in "safer sex" are the greatest threats to sexual wellbeing. To refrain from enjoyable, joyful and pleasurable, but risky, sexual behaviors is associated with feelings of loss, suffering, grief, and rage. Feelings of being plague-stricken, not attractive any longer, and not having the right to a sex life may also contribute to the threat of sexual wellbeing. Another threat is the HIV-infection and its potential impact on sexual desire and/or sexual functioning. Among Swedish HIV-carriers there is a legal threat as well. The Swedish Communicable Diseases Act requires disclosure of one's HIV-seropositivity as well as condom use when practicing anal, vaginal, or oral intercourse.

EXISTENTIAL VERSUS NEUROTIC ANXIETY

Various kinds of anxiety reactions can be evoked within the HIV-carrier as a response to the above mentioned threats and worries. They can be of an existential as well as of a neurotic character.

The nucleus of all anxiety is the fear of being alone, separated, and helpless and it originates from the baby's experiences of loss, aloneness, and helplessness. These experiences will eventually constitute a psychological basis for adult life-crisis. Being in a life crisis, experiencing its related guilt reactions, the individual gets in touch with his/her existential anxiety. It is a reflection of insight into the inescapable limitations of existence and the individual's aloneness and vulnerability (Wikström, 1990). The child's separation anxiety corresponds to the adult's experience of a total helplessness towards universal mortality. Everything will cease and the individual will be brought inexorably towards the final separation, death.

Death is the most obvious given of our existence (Yalom, 1980). We exist now, but death will come and there is no escape from it. We respond to this terrible truth with conscious and unconscious fear. The fear of death is of such magnitude that we develop various defense mechanisms in order to cope with it.

Usually when we talk about death fear we actually refer to fears *related* to death (Kastenbaum, 1972) such as the event of dying and/or what comes after death (Choren, 1964). From an existential point of view, however, ceasing to be is the central fear of death (Yalom, 1980). But death is not the only ultimate concern that is an inescapable part of our existence in the world. Freedom, isolation, and meaninglessness are also givens of existence with which we are confronted (Yalom, 1980).

Freedom, in its existential sense, refers to each individual's entire responsibility for his or her own world, life design, choices, and actions.

Existential isolation indicates our fundamental isolation, i.e., each of us enters existence alone and must depart from it alone. In other words, there is no "stand in" for my death, no one can die my death for me.

Finally, the ultimate concern of *meaninglessness*. If we must die, if we must constitute our own world, if we are ultimately alone, then what meaning does life have? Why do we live? And how shall we live? Yalom (1980) emphasizes that the human being is a meaning-seeking creature who is thrown into a universe that has no known meaning. Thus, each of us has to construct our own meanings in life.

Existential anxiety is thus an anxiety reaction to the inescapability of the ultimate concerns. Neurotic anxiety on the other hand is generated from unconscious, internal, repressed conflicts. There is, however, a link between the two: "The existential anxiety of death, personal responsibility, guilt, and questions about the meaning of life can be reinforced, colored, and intermittently exceeded by a non-worked through internal conflict from the first years of life. Worries of annihilation, that are embedded in the consciousness of one's own death, can be affected unproportionately strong by early losses and non-healed griefs'' (pp. 82-83, Wikström, 1990).

PSYCHOLOGICAL DYSFUNCTIONING

Given the tremendous worries of eventually developing life-threatening complications together with the worries of social and sexual existences, it is not surprising that HIV-carriers can suffer virtually any form of stress-related psychological dysfunctioning. It should be noted that the vast majority of HIV-related psychological research has been conducted among homosexual men.

Examples of the most commonly reported dysfunctions are acute stress reactions (World Health Organization, 1988, 1990; Fenton et al. 1987; Miller, 1987; Nichols, 1985), adjustment disorders (World Health Organization, 1990) and clinical depression (Zecca Mansueto & Moroni, 1991; Calalan, 1988; Ostrow et al., 1986; Dilley et al., 1985; Perry et al., 1984). Data indicate that HIV-seropositive women score higher on depression and psychological distress in general than do their male counterparts (Bromberg et al., 1991; Carey et al., 1991). Another study (Murphy et al., 1991) identified the following predictors of depression among homosexual HIV-carriers: perception of fewer social supports and not feeling needed as a source of support; more severe illness; and lower internal locus of control.

It is, however, most important to distinguish psychological reactions to HIV infection from the symptoms arising out of central nervous system involvement (e.g., confusional states, chronic impairment in intellectual functioning). It is often difficult to make this distinction, as mood disturbances or psychotic features are often the presenting symptoms of an organic brain syndrome (Miller and Riccio, 1990).

Associated with depression is the increased risk of suicidal planning and activity among HIV-seropositive persons (Gala et al., 1989; Marzuk et al., 1988). However, an earlier psychiatric history and a history of attempted suicide are better predictors of current suicidal activity than a diagnosis of HIV infection (Gala et al., 1989). These data are in line with a study focusing on homosexual long term survivors with AIDS (Remien et al., 1991). In the absence of a past suicide attempt, a diagnosis of AIDS alone did not appear to lead to an increased risk for suicide in this cohort. Suicidal responses have also followed where HIV-positive results have been identified without pre-test counseling or without consent (Miller et al., 1986). A recent study (Rundell et al., 1988) identified the following predictive factors of suicidal attempts among HIV-infected USAF personnel: (1) multiple psychosocial stresses; (2) perceived social isolation; (3) perceiving oneself as a victim; (4) reliance on denial as the central and only defense; (5) substance abuse; (6) perceived unavailable social support and (7) earlier history of psychiatric illness.

Acute psychotic disorders and paranoid disorders are rarely reported within the HIV-positive population of Center for Disease Control (CDC) classification II and III (CDC, 1986). But a number of reports (Buhrich et al., 1988; Halstead et al., 1988; Jones, 1987; Vogel-Scibilia et al., 1988) have documented psychoses within CDC classification IV.

The important mediating role of social support in psychological wellbeing among HIV-carriers is clearly demonstrated in various studies (Reisbeck et al., 1991; Ostrow et al. 1991; Hays, 1990; Straits et al., 1990; Zick & Temoshok, 1990; Wolcott et al., 1986). Other studies have focused on social variables such as coping styles, attributional tendencies and internalized homophobia among homo- and bisexual men and their impact on psychological wellbeing. Data show that avoidant coping styles are associated with greater distress (e.g., anxiety, depression) and lower self-esteem (Namir et al., 1990, Wolf et al., 1991; Weimer et al., 1991), sexual dysfunctions and psychosomatic symptoms (Nilsson Schönnesson, 1991), and lower social support (Namir et al., 1990, Wolf et al., 1991; Weimer et al., 1991). Active-behavioral coping styles, on the other hand, appear to be related to enhanced mood and greater perceived social support (Namir et al., 1990, Wolf et al., 1991).

Nicholson and Long (1990) studied predictors of various coping strategies. They found in their HIV-positive homosexual men that greater internalized homophobia and less self-esteem predicted avoidant coping, whereas less homophobia and less time since diagnosis predicted proactive coping (seeking social support, planful problem solving).

A positive attitude toward homosexuality has been shown to correlate positively with lower emotional distress in AIDS patients (Wolcott et al., 1986). Greater time since diagnosis, less avoidant coping, less homophobia, and greater self-esteem predicted better mood state (Nicholson and Long, 1990). Self-blame with respect to infection and health improvement has been associated with increased emotional distress in gay men with AIDS (Moulton et al., 1987).

Scattered case reports (Lippert, 1986; Nurnberg et al., 1984; Polan et al., 1985) have documented loss of sexual desire and sexual dysfunctions among HIV-carriers. That sexual functioning should be affected by the HIV-infection is quite plausible for many reasons: an individual's emotional reaction to her/his HIV-diagnosis and/or its related symptoms and diseases or to the HIV-epidemic in general, psychological dysfunctioning, psychiatric states, possible neurological effects of this neurotropic virus, the systemic effects of advanced stages of HIV disease, and the experimental medication used for the treatment of HIV-related symptoms and diseases (Meyer-Bahlburg et al., 1991).

However, with one exception, no systematic studies of the extent of sexual dysfunctions or other sexual problems in HIV-carriers in various stages of the disease have been undertaken. Meyer-Bahlburg and his colleagues (1991) assessed sexual functioning in a sample of HIV-positive and HIV-negative homo- and bisexual men and correlated their findings with symptoms and signs of HIV-disease progression. The HIV-carriers reported experiencing significantly more frequent problems with sexual interest, pleasure, and erection, but not with orgasmic functioning. None of the sexual problems were, however, correlated with HIV-related symptoms and/or diseases.

Siegel and Krauss (1991) have pointed out, that despite a small but growing body of empirical and clinical literature on psychosocial adaptation to HIV, there have been no published studies that attempt to identify the challenges of living daily with HIV-infection in CDC classification I-III. In their study they examined the challenges of daily living faced by seropositive homosexual men. The following three major adaptive challenges were identified: dealing with the possibility of a curtailed lifespan, dealing with reactions to a stigmatizing disease, and developing strategies for maintaining physical and emotional health.

HIV-ADAPTATION PROCESSES

Given the threats of and worries about social, physical, and sexual existences, and their related emotional reactions, the HIV-carrier is confronted with the great challenge of trying to cope with, adapt to, and to learn to live with her/his chronic HIV-infection. To learn to live with HIV-infection is a life-long adaptation-process. It is like a movie, where some scenes are sometimes frozen for a longer or shorter time. The scenes may flourish in light, hope, and confidence or darkness, hopelessness, and despair. But regardless of "lightness," there is always an undercurrent of deep emotional suffering.

In describing psychological processes operating in HIV-carriers the most common theoretical models being used are the five-stage model of grief (Kubler-Ross, 1969) or similar stage-crisis models. My clinical and scientific work with homosexual HIV-carriers have made me critical in using these stage-crisis models. Kubler-Ross's model, for example, is aimed at describing the emotional reactions and the coming to terms with dying and death. Other stage-crisis models focus on mainly the acute phase of a crisis, i.e., emotional reactions to a disease diagnosis, and the development of restoring the psychological equilibrium. Bearing in mind that HIV-infection is characterized by a long period of latency or slow progression in which the HIV-carrier may be confronted with various HIV-related worries/threats, it is questionable whether these models are appropriate in describing and analyzing the adaptation process of HIV-carriers. The crisis models have also a tendency to give the impression of a "right" or "normal" way to react. For those HIV-carriers who do not perceive that they are going through the stages in the right order, feelings of guilt or being abnormal may be evoked.

Instead of stage-models, I would like to suggest a model based upon the concept of *adaptation*. Although the model is based upon clinical experiences from homosexual HIV-carriers, it is not unlikely that the theoretical model may be applicable to HIV-carriers in general.

In the case of HIV, it is not only a question of adapting to psychological processes, but also to practical and social circumstances. "Adaptation" does not refer to a normative concept, but to a subjective adaptation constituted by the individual's access to her/his psychological and social resources. Examples of intrapersonal resources are defense mechanisms, coping style, and coping strategy. Interpersonal resources refer to social networks and social supports. The adaptation process is a process of change, in which the aim is to become better prepared to deal with current life conditions. In the course of the adaptation-process, the individual develops adaptation-strategies by means of her/his intrapersonal and interpersonal resources.

It is here suggested that these adaptation-strategies are changeable, depending upon circumstances, conditions, and earlier experiences. The aim of a given adaptation strategy is to minimize experiences of mental suffering, to cope with the uncertainty associated with the HIV-infection, and to provide the individual with a feeling of control, thus achieving–at least temporarily–a psychological well-being.

CONCLUSION

HIV-infection, and all its medical, psychological, social and economic ramifications, creates enormous suffering among HIV-carriers, but also among partners, relatives, friends, and health care workers. But HIV can also be looked upon as a challenge, regardless of HIV-status. From my perspective, HIV infection is a challenge of our modes of existing in this world.

Martin Heidegger (1962) believed that there are two fundamental modes of existing in the world: (1) *a state of forgetfulness of being,* or (2) *a state of mindfulness of being.* Ordinarily we live in the first state, in which we surrender ourselves to a concern about the *way* things are. Heidegger means that the state of forgetfulness of being is a mode in which one is unaware of one's authorship of one's life and world. In the state of mindfulness of being, one marvels *that* things are. In this mode one remains mindful of the fragility of being and of one's responsibility for one's own being. In order to be able to live life in such an authentic fashion, we have to integrate the *idea* of death. Rather than sentence us to existences of terror or bleak pessimism, the idea of death acts as a catalyst to plunge us into more authentic life modes, and it enhances our pleasure in the living of life (Heidegger, 1962).

REFERENCES

Albert, E. (1986). Illness and Deviance: The Response of the Press to AIDS. Pp. 163-178 in Feldman, D.A. & Johnson, T.M. (Eds.) *The Social Dimensions of AIDS. Method and Theory.* New York: Praeger.

Bromberg, J., Grijalva, K., Skurnick, J., Cordell, J., Wan, J., Cornell, R., & Louria, D. (1991). Psychological differences between HIV+ women and HIV+ men in discordant couples: A report from the heterosexual HIV transmission study (HATS). VII *International Conference on Aids, Firenze, Abstract. W.D. 4128.*

Buhrich, N., Cooper, D.A., & Freed, E. (1988). HIV-infection associated with symptoms indistinguishable from functional psychosis. *British Journal of Psychiatry,* 152,649-653.

Carey, M.A., Jenkins, R.A., Brown, G.K., & Temoshok, L. (1991). Gender differences in psychological functioning in early stage HIV. VII *International Conference on Aids, Firenze, Abstract. M.D. 4230.*

Catalan, J. (1988). Psychosocial and neuropsychiatric aspects of HIV infection: review of their extent and implications for psychiatry. *J of Psychosom Res* 32,237-248.

Choren, J. (1964). *Modern Man and Mortality.* New York: MacMillan.

Dilley, J.W., Ochitill, H.N., Perl, M., & Volberding, P. (1985). Findings in psychiatric consultations with patients with acquired immune deficiency syndrome. *Am J Psychiatry,* 142,82-86.

Fenton, T.W. (1986). AIDS-related psychiatric disorder. *Br J Psychiatry,* 151,579-588.

Gala, C., Merkin, S., Pergeuni, A. (1989). Psychiatric history among homosexuals and drug addicts infected with HIV. V *International Conference on AIDS, Montreal, Abstract. W.B.P. 216.*

Halstead, S., Riccio, M., Harlow, P., Oretti, R., & Thompson, C. (1988). Psychosis associated with HIV infection. *British Journal of Psychiatry,* 153,618-623.

Hays, R.B., Chauncey, S., & Tobey, L.A. (1990). The social support networks of gay men with AIDS. *Journ Commun Psycho,* 18,374-385.

Heidegger, M. (1962). *Being and Time.* New York: Harper & Row.

Jones, H.G. (1987). HIV and onset of schizophrenia. *Lancet,* i, 982.

Kastenbaum, R. and Aisenberg, R. (1972). *Psychology of Death.* New York: Springer.

Kubler-Ross, E. (1969). *On death and dying.* London: MacMillan.

Lippert, G.P. (1986). Excessive concern about AIDS in two bisexual men. *Canadian Journal of Psychiatry,* 31,63-65.

Marzuk, P.M., Tierney, H., & Tardiff, K. (1988). Increased risk of suicide in persons with AIDS. *JAMA,* 259,1333-1337.

Meyer-Bahlburg, H., Exner, T.M., Lorenz, G., Gruen, R.S., Gorman, J.M., & Ehrhardt, A.A. (1991). Sexual risk behavior, sexual functioning, and HIV-disease progression in gay men. *The Journal of Sex Research,* 28,3-27.

Miller, D. & M. Riccio (1990). Editorial Review: Non-organic psychiatric and psychosocial syndromes associated with HIV-1 infection and disease. AIDS, 4,381-388.

Miller, D., Jeffries, D.J, Grenn, J., Harris, J.R.W, & Pinching, A.J. (1986). HTLV-III:should testing ever be routine? *British Medical Journal*, 292,941-943.

Miller, D. (1987). *Living with AIDS and HIV*. London: Macmillan Press.

Moulton, J., Sweet, D., & Temoshok, L. (1990). Understanding attributions and health behavior changes in AIDS and ARC: Implications for interventions. Pp. 191-200 in L. Temoshok & A. Baum (1990) *Psychosocial Perspectives on AIDS. Etiology, Prevention, and Treatment*. New Jersey: Lawrence Erlbaum Ass.

Murphy, D., Kelley, J.A., Brasfield, T., Koob, J., Bahr, R., & St Lawrence, J. (1991). Predictors of depression among persons with HIV infection. *VII International Conference on AIDS, Firenze, Abstract. W.D. 4276*.

Namir, S., Wolcott, D., Fawsey, F. & Alumbaugh, M. (1990). Implications of different strategies for coping with AIDS. Pp. 173-190 in L. Temoshok & A. Baum (1990) *Psychosocial Perspectives on AIDS. Etiology, Prevention, and Treatment*. New Jersey: Lawrence Erlbaum Ass.

Nichols, SE. (1986). An overview of the psychological and social reactions to AIDS. In *Acquired Immunodeficiency Syndrome: International Conference on AIDS, Paris, 23-25 June 1986* edited by Gluckman, J.C. & Vilmer, E. Paris: Elsevier, p. 262.

Nicholson, W.D. & Long, B.C. (1990). Self-Esteem, Social Support, Internalized Homophobia, and Coping Strategies of HIV+ Gay Men. *Journ Consult and Clin Psychol*, 58,873-876.

Nilsson Schönnesson, L. (1991). *Coping styles and psychological wellbeing among HIV-positive homosexual men*. Stockholm: Unpublished paper.

Nilsson Schönnesson, L. (1991). *Stress, adaptation, and psychological wellbeing of homosexual HIV-carriers*. Stockholm: Unpublished paper.

Nurnberg, H.G., Prudic, J., Fiori, M., & Freedman, E.P. (1984). Psychopathology complicating Acquired Immune Deficiency Syndrome (AIDS). *American Journal of Psychiatry*, 141,95-96.

Ostrow, D.G., Whitaker, R.E.D., Fraiser, K., Cohen, C., Fisher, E. et al. (1991). Racial differences in social support and mental health in men with HIV-infection: a pilot study. *AIDS Care*, 3,55-62.

Ostrow, D.G., Joseph, J., & Monjan, A. (1986). Psychosocial aspects of AIDS risk. *Psychopharmacol Bull.*, 22,678-683.

Perry, SW. & Tross, S. (1984). Psychiatric problems of AIDS in-patients at the New York Hospital: a preliminary report. *Public Health Rep.*, 99,200-205.

Polan, H.J., Hellerstein, D., & Anchin, J. (1985). Impact of AIDS-related cases on an inpatient therapeutic milieu. *Hospital and Community Psychiatry*, 36,173-176.

Remien, R., Rabkin, J., Katoff, L., & Williams, J. (1991). Suicidality and psychological outlook in long term survivors of AIDS. *VII International Conference on AIDS, Firenze, Abstract. M.D. 105*.

Rundell, J., Thomason, J., Zajac, R., & Beatty, R. (1988). Psychiatric diagnosis and attempted suicide (AS) in HIV-infected USAF personnel. *IV International Conference on AIDS, Stockholm, Abstract. 8585.*

Siegel, K. & Krauss, B.J. (1991). Living with HIV infection: Adaptive Tasks of Seropositive Gay Men. *Journal of Health and Social Behavior*, 32,17-32.

Straits, K., Temoshok, L., & Zich, J. (1990). A cross-cultural comparison of psychosocial responses to having AIDS and related conditions in London and San Francisco. Pp. 139-166 in L. Temoshok & A. Baum (1990) *Psychosocial Perspectives on AIDS. Etiology, Prevention, and Treatment.* New Jersey: Lawrence Erlbaum Ass.

Vogel-Scibilia, S.E., Mulsant, B.H., & Keshavab, M.S. (1988). HIV infection presenting as psychosis: a critique. *Acta Psychitr. Scand.*, 78,652-656.

Weimer, E., Clement. U., & Nilsson Schönnesson, L. (1991). Depressive Reaktionen und psychische Verarbeitung bei HIV-positiven homosexuellen Männern. *Psychotherapy, Psychosomatik, Medicine Psychologie*, 41,107-114.

Wikström, O. (1990). *Den outgrundliga människan. Livsfrågor, psykoterapi och själavård.* Stockholm: Natur och Kultur.

Wolcott, D., Namir, S., et al. (1986). Illness concerns, attitudes towards homosexuality, and social support in gay men with AIDS. *General Hospital Psychiatry*, 8,395-403.

Wolf, T.M., Balson, P.M., Morse, E.V., Simon, P.M., Williams, M.H. et al. (1991). Relationship of coping style to affective state and perceived social support in asymptomatic and symptomatic HIV-infected persons: Implications for clinical management. *Journ Clin Psych*, 52,171-173.

World Health Organization (1988). *Report of the Consultation on the Neuropsychiatric Aspects of HIV Infection.* Geneva: WHO, 14-17 March, 1988.

World Health Organization (1990). *ICD-10 Chapter V: Mental and Behavioural Disorders (Draft).* February 1990.

Yalom, I.D. (1980). *Existential Psychotherapy.* New York: Basic Books.

Zecca Mansueto, G. & Moroni, P. (1991). Psychological follow-up of haemophilic patients with HIV infection. *VII International Conference on AIDS, Firenze, Abstract. W.D. 4213.*

Zich, J., & Temoshok, L. (1990) Perceptions of social support, distress and hopelessness in men with AIDS and ARC: clinical implication. Pp. 201-228 in L. Temoshok & A, Baum (1990) *Psychosocial Perspectives on AIDS. Etiology, Prevention, and Treatment.* New Jersey: Lawrence Erlbaum Ass.

Shifts in Meaning, Purpose, and Values Following a Diagnosis of Human Immunodeficiency Virus (HIV) Infection Among Gay Men

Susan Schaefer, PhD
Eli Coleman, PhD

SUMMARY. Twenty gay men who were HIV infected were interviewed and a qualitative methodology was utilized to understand how they found meaning, purpose and value in their lives as they confronted a life-threatening illness. The authors examined six areas of potential meaning derived deductively from thanatology literature and inductively from piloting procedures: (1) relationships (intimacy with others); (2) self-discovery; (3) spiritual fulfillment; (4) acquiring knowledge; (5) aesthetic appreciation/involvement; and (6) contributing to others or society. Nearly all of the participants (85%) reported that their overall sense of meaning, purpose and value had

Susan Schaefer is in private practice in Minneapolis, MN. Eli Coleman is Director and Associate Professor, Program in Human Sexuality, Department of Family Practice and Community Health, University of Minnesota Medical School. Requests for reprints may be sent to the second author at the Program in Human Sexuality, 1300 South 2nd Street, Suite 180, Minneapolis, MN 55454.

This paper was part of a larger study which was completed as part of the requirements for a doctoral dissertation at Saybrook University, San Francisco, CA. This research was conducted at the HIV Clinic at the University of Minnesota Hospitals and Clinic. The authors would like to thank Dr. Frank Rhame, the director of this clinic, for his assistance in helping us identify subjects for this research as well as his helpful suggestions and comments. They would also like to thank Anne Marie Ford, a counselor at the clinic, who helped id assisted with pilot interviews. This research was funded thro seling Center which has received funds from the Thorpe Foun cy Foundation. The authors are most grateful to the participa their time, energy, and insight into the psychological proces:

changed since being diagnosed seropositive. The greatest number of this subgroup reported that a positive change had occurred. Three persons (15%) felt their HIV status adversely affected their sense of meaning of life. The factor most likely to account for the positive shifts in meaning came from the realization that their time of living was limited. Relationships brought the greatest sense of meaning, purpose and value. Religion or a spiritual life was the category of meaning which provided the least comfort. A number of men who were no longer able to work at their jobs turned to artistic expression and volunteerism for fulfillment. This information should be helpful to HIV-infected individuals and to caregivers who wish to assist them.

INTRODUCTION

Following the first reported cases of HIV/AIDS in 1981 came reports of the disease's shattering psychological ramifications (Morin and Batchelor, 1984; Malyon, 1984; and Nichols, 1984). These preliminary reports, based on clinical observations and anecdotal information, emphasized that although persons with HIV/AIDS typically felt their medical needs were being adequately addressed, their psychological needs were being overlooked. In describing the psychological reactions to HIV/AIDS, nearly all of the literature to date has used the five stage model of grief described by Kubler-Ross (1969).

The diagnosis of HIV/AIDS presents a very complicated clinical picture to health care providers both medically and psychologically. Given the fact that this disease primarily affects young adults in the United States (aged 20-40), the more gradual developmental and existential process of coming to grips with mortality and the meaning of life (often occurring in later years) must necessarily be encapsulated into a much shorter period of time. The attempt to find a sense of purpose and personal significance in the face of catastrophic disease is perhaps the greatest challenge in coping with this disease. The significant increase in suicide rates among persons with AIDS (36 times greater than matched controls [Marzuk, Tierney, Tardiff, Gross, Morgan, Hsu, and Mann, 1988]) in part suggests the tremendous struggle to discover meaning and purpose during the course of this disease.

Through her early work with dying patients, Kubler-Ross has shown that it is possible to find purpose and psychological resolution to the existential crises produced by terminal illness. However, critics have stated that the Kubler-Ross model is of "limited usefulness in describing reactions to the HIV infection" (Ross, Tebble and Viliunas, 1989). In spite of this criticism, these researchers have nonetheless gone on to use aspects of this model in their own work.

With nearly all of the HIV/AIDS psychological adjustment literature based on anecdotal and clinical reports, the need for systematic studies designed to assess psychological aspects of adaptation to HIV/AIDS was clear (Batchelor, 1984).

In defining the direction scientifically valid and community relevant research on psychosocial aspects of AIDS should take, Joseph and colleagues stated the following: "We believe that any serious effort to study the impact of AIDS on gay men must attempt to understand the phenomenology of the crisis from the perspective of those exposed to it." (Joseph, Emmons, Kessler, Wortman, O'Brien, Hocker & Schaefer, 1984, p. 1297).

By systematically studying psychological aspects of adaptation to HIV/AIDS, this research has attempted to circumvent one of the primary criticisms of earlier reports: namely, that findings were based on anecdotal reports alone. Through phenomenological analysis, this study examines HIV-seropositive gay men's subjective experience of meaning, purpose and value in their lives while confronting this catastrophic disease.

METHODS

Subjects

The charts of 150 patients referred to the HIV clinic at the University of Minnesota were examined in search of an appropriate sample of 20 for this study. Beginning March 1, 1990, all patients whose charts were active, as well as those presenting to the clinic for the first time following that date, were reviewed. In order to increase homogeneity of the sample, the following criteria were established in selecting subjects for this study:

1. Self-identified gay males
2. Caucasian
3. Between the ages of 20-55
4. Diagnosed seropositive
5. U.S. citizen
6. High school (or beyond) education.

Once potential subjects meeting the above criteria were identified, they were handed a letter of introduction, given a brief description of this study and their participation was requested. Persons agreeing to participate in the study were then given a copy of the informed consent agreement to review and sign. The ages of the subjects in this study can be viewed in Table 1.

Education. Eighty percent of the sample had some technical training or partial college education following their high school education and diploma. Twenty percent of persons in this sample completed a college education, with one person having received his masters degree.

Income and Occupation. Thirty percent of the participants were supporting themselves through social security disability income or other governmental funding provided for persons with catastrophic illness. Their income ranged from $4,872 to $11,400 per year, with additional subsidies for housing, food allowances and medical care. Among those employed (70%), incomes ranged from $10,500 to $50,000 with an average income of $25,785. Occupations were scattered evenly among five primary occupational categories: service, technical, management, small business owner/operator, and professional.

HIV Status. Eight (40%) of the sample had met criteria for a diagnosis of AIDS. Four (20%) were unaware of whether they technically met the guidelines for AIDS. The remaining eight (40%) were seropositive with no diagnosis of AIDS.

The Interview

This study was part of a larger interview study which assessed stressful life events associated with the diagnosis and progression

Table 1

Participant's Ages

Age Category	Number	Percent
21-25	1	5
26-30	3	15
31-35	4	20
36-40	9	45
41-45	1	5
46-50	0	0
51-55	2	10

Age Range: 23-53   Median Age: 36

of HIV and determined what types of support were or would have been most helpful in managing those stressors. A semi-structured interview was used which ranged between 1 to 3 1/4 hours in length. A portion of the interview tapped six areas of potential meaning, purpose or value of life derived deductively from thanatology literature and inductively from piloting procedures: (1) relationships (intimacy with others); (2) self-discovery; (3) spiritual fulfillment; (4) acquiring knowledge; (5) aesthetic appreciation/involvement; and (6) contributing to others or society. The questionnaire also included a number of open-ended questions which offered opportunities for the participant to discuss issues beyond the predetermined categories (see Appendix).

Data Analysis

Qualitative data obtained from the interviews were assessed through thematic content analyses. This reflective abstractive approach (Inhelder and Piaget, 1958) was used to analyze the shared meanings contained in the interviews. This was accomplished through grouping similar statements into content groups and abstracting the information until primary categories were defined and essential meanings (or *meaning units* as they are referred to in phenomenological literature) emerged through the interviewing process. In keeping with Lofland and Lofland's (1984) directive that meanings are best "seen" and analyzed when one assumes a "reality constructionist" stance, this theoretical framework was assumed throughout the research. The reality constructionist stance holds that meanings are not inherent in reality but are imputed by humans.

Giorgi (1989), summarized the essential methodological steps required for qualitative data analysis in this way: (1) reading the material; (2) breaking the material into parts; (3) making sense of the parts through a disciplined or professional way; and (4) reintegration of the parts.

The computer software program *Hyperqual* (Padilla, 1989) was used to systematize this process of qualitative data analysis. This program consists of four stacks which store and organize data derived from interview content. These stacks hold formatted cards which are reproduced as needed to store as much data as a particular interview or collection of interviews generates. Data entered onto these cards, which are identified as meaningful data *chunks*, are highlighted and sent through identifier *buttons* to specific output files. These files become part of an emerging account, constructed by the analyst interacting with the phenomenon under study. During the preliminary analysis, it is not necessary to categorize or codify data. Thematically related text segments can be collated or *chunked* in an output file. Once the analyst is ready to group data chunks together, individual codes called *tags* are attached to the text segments comprising these meaningful data chunks. The data chunks are then sent to new stacks where further refinement of the chunking and coding process takes place. The sorted stacks of text can easily be scanned, called up and printed out, allowing the analyst to add, change, or delete codes as data chunks are further grouped according to an emerging pattern or account. This software program does not predetermine the process by which data is ultimately analyzed, nor does it require the data to be pre-structured, allowing for maximal flexibility in the data analysis.

RESULTS

Nearly all of the participants (85%) reported that their overall sense of meaning, purpose and value had changed since being diagnosed seropositive. The greatest number of this subgroup reported a positive change, typically noting that they no longer took life for granted. They reported squeezing more life out of each day by taking advantage of opportunities instead of waiting, by living life more consciously with greater attention to detail, and by letting go of petty concerns sooner.

The factor most likely to account for the positive shifts in meaning came from the simple realization that their time of living was limited; therefore, they felt that there was no time to waste. The potential terminality of the disease was an ongoing reminder of mortality to the men, many of whom were reminded and re-reminded of it as they buried their past partners and friends.

The experience of being seropositive brought a change in general outlook or philosophy towards life to nearly all the participants (90%). For most it brought a sense of urgency to set about doing what they really wanted to do in life, and a richness and intensification of their life experiences.

Another dynamic which many participants described in different ways, was the development of a stronger inner locus of control. Whether it showed up in decisions to give up addictions (alcohol, nicotine), the commitment to a regular exercise program or a greater focus on what truly made them happy in their work and personal life, a significant number of men in this sample described the process of turning inward rather than outward for direction in their lives.

A number of people were quite specific in describing the rewards that such a change in outlook brought them. One man stated he looked on his illness as a blessing, there to teach him. As a result of being HIV positive, he stated he had developed a much greater appreciation for strangers, friends, family, work, nature and life itself. He also reported becoming much less judgmental of others. The general tone of his comments were echoed throughout the interviews.

Three persons (15%) felt their HIV status adversely affected their sense of meaning of life. These subjects experienced bouts of depression and low self-esteem and attributed this negative shift to cultural prejudice about homosexuality and HIV-infected individuals and lack of acceptance and compassion by others in their lives.

One of these three men had made two serious suicide attempts and was hospitalized a third time for suicidal intent. He stated that a positive sense of meaning, purpose or value was fleeting; on a given day he might or might not feel positively. At the time he was being interviewed, he had decided he would not make any further attempts on his life because he had recently learned from his primary physician that he was the longest surviving AIDS patient his doctor had treated and he stated it simply wasn't fair to have had his doctor work for years to keep him alive only for him to kill himself. Another man who was grieving many losses in his life stated: "Lately there hasn't been a purpose to life, with the loss of work, partner and family. Sometimes I just don't think there is meaning."

Relationships

Relationships brought the greatest sense of meaning, purpose and value to participants. Ninety percent (18) of the men stressed the importance of relationships in their lives. The remaining two individuals were more noncommittal in response to this question, saying they either weren't sure or relationships were too hard to come by for them to give a more detailed answer.

One man remarked that during the course of his illness, developing and maintaining relationships took on ever greater meaning to him. As other avenues for the experience of meaning closed down with the illness, relationships could remain a constant, though expressed differently over time. Partners, friends, children, grandchildren and other family members were all mentioned in this category.

Though not implied in the pre-existing relationship category, the open-ended question of meaning of life indicated that pets should be considered part of the category of relationships. A quarter of the participants discussed the significant role that pets played in their lives. One man who lived alone credited his dog with indirectly saving his life. During a particularly vegetative depression, he was having difficulty getting out of bed. He stated that there were days in which the only reason he had to get up was to walk or feed his dog. Without the responsibility of caring for his dog, he was not sure he would still be alive. One man who had been advised to give up his cats (due to the diseases they carry) as well as dairy products (due to bacteria which could put him at risk for infection) decided that a life without cats and ice cream was no life at all, and continued to enjoy both.

Fifty percent of the participants were not in a sexually committed relationship although many of these men expressed a desire for such. These men stated they wanted to date, but were fearful of having to tell a prospective partner that they were seropositive. These men responded with great enthusiasm about pursuing dating when told that nearly every other participant interviewed indicated that the one thing which would make it easier for them to date, would be to find out that the other person was seropositive as well.

Spiritual Fulfillment

Whereas relationships with other persons proved to be one of the most important areas of meaning for the men in this study group, religion or a spiritual life was the category of meaning which provided the least comfort of any of the six major areas surveyed. To many, beyond not providing comfort, it proved to be disappointing or disturbing.

One-fourth of the men clearly felt no affiliation and no ability to draw on a sense of strength or connection in the area of spirituality. Many more were dominated by feelings of disenfranchisement and were struggling to develop or evolve a spiritual presence in their lives. A number of men described the difficulty they had in getting beyond the stance of mainstream religions whose philosophy towards homosexuality is best summed up as "love the sinner, hate the sin." They perceived it as outrageous hypocrisy that on the one hand, many of the churches they tried to get involved with would provide pastoral care or volunteer services to people with HIV/AIDS while prevailing attitudes of church doctrine were patronizing or even deploring of homosexuality.

Of the 40% who did feel a connection with a higher power, none reported attending church regularly. Instead, spirituality in their lives was nurtured through artistic expression, meditation, visualization and the general feeling of being part of the great mystery of life. In describing their religious connection, most in the group adopted religious viewpoints and modes of expression which are best characterized as Buddhist in theological content and context. A few spoke of their relationship with a higher power in Christian terminology. Other religious philosophies were not as clearly identifiable.

Self Discovery

Self growth or the development of insights and understanding about themselves was a very significant source of meaning and value to many of the participants. Responses suggested that confronting a catastrophic illness dramatically heightens one's awareness of mortality. One man graphically described the omnipresence of death as an internal pulsating voice, chanting "AIDS, AIDS, AIDS" relentlessly and incessantly during his waking hours.

This feeling of time running out advanced their developmental process well beyond chronological years, with many feeling developmentally kindred to the aged. Some of these men described this in terms of rapid maturing, with an accompanying change of values which were less materialistic; others defined it as becoming less achievement oriented and outer directed and more introspective and inner focused. Still others frankly stated that they related to the elderly in thoughts, feelings and life issues.

Many of the men surveyed considered their change in focus one of the rewards of their illness. They were quite emphatic about how important a change in direction had become in terms of providing more meaning and connection in their lives. One man described how much he valued living alone because it afforded him more time for self-reflection.

Acquiring Knowledge

Three-quarters of the participants indicated that their ability to acquire information and skills brought them a sense of meaning, purpose or value. Mastering skills was identified as important to many men who described creating or building things as giving them a sense of value. One man clearly stated that the development of his abilities was tied to his self-esteem. For the majority of men who endorsed this meaning category, the knowledge they referred to had little to do with academic learning. Instead it centered more on knowledge which enabled them to acquire practical information or skills (e.g., learning about the medical aspects of managing their disease, learning how to express themselves artistically). This search for practical knowledge appeared to be a priority before acquiring their seropositive states, however became intensified after their diagnosis of HIV/AIDS.

Aesthetic Appreciation/Involvement

The original category of Aesthetic Appreciation was redefined to include participatory forms of aesthetic endeavors after it became apparent through the interviews that artistic expression grew in its importance to the respondents over the course of their disease. As their illness progressed, avenues of meaning, purpose and value often needed to be redefined as physical limitations interfered with previous ones, particularly those related to work. A number of men who were no longer able to work at their jobs turned to artistic expression for fulfillment.

They accomplished this through writing short-stories, journaling about their experience of living with HIV/AIDS, writing poetry and making films to tell their stories. For two men in the sample, artistic expression was their life's work. One man was a professional dancer, another a very successful interior designer who referred to his most creative works as his memorials, the legacy he would leave behind to mark his existence. One of these men reported an urgency of expression, indicating he would die quickly if he could not create. He considered it as necessary as breathing.

Ninety percent (18) of the men described artistic appreciation and involvement as a source of meaning, purpose or value in their lives. Those persons who valued it more from a spectator vantage point than that of a participator, described the arts as motivating them, spurring their own creativity and serving as a source of comfort, richness and inspiration in life. One man noted that listening to music was an especially powerful form of connection and meaning to him. For him, it was a link to some of his best friends who had died of AIDS before him, many of whom were female impersonators. By replaying songs these friends used in their stage acts, he felt carried back to them. During these times he would converse with them and find solace in their revealing to him (he reports) directions they felt he should take in his life.

Most often, these creative vehicles of expression were being used to communicate personal feelings and truths about the experience of living with the exigencies of a life-threatening disease. At times these creative expressions were shared with no one; at other times, they were made public, as in the case of one man who was making a film about men with a seropositive diagnosis who were living well over a span of many years. Whether these expressions remained private reflections or were translated into public performances, their value to participants was immeasurable.

Contributing to Others or Society

Ninety percent (18) of the participants designated this category as an important source of meaning in their lives. Beyond their willingness to contribute to this study, a number of the participants found value through participation in other research studies devoted to the study of HIV/AIDS. One man was particularly determined to offer himself as a subject in anything HIV/AIDS-related, feeling as though it was part of his current mission in life. He stated: "I, by rights, shouldn't be here. It's been five years. Five years ago I thought I had a year. Who knows, maybe I'll be here until they have a cure." Others found different arenas for contributing to HIV/AIDS related causes, through political activism, educating others about safer sex, volunteering for social service agencies which cater to persons with HIV/AIDS or serving as caregivers to persons with AIDS. One man indicated that he planned to sign up with a local AIDS organization to serve as a caregiver in advance of his own need for custodial care, so he wouldn't feel guilty when the time eventually came for his own need for it. Beyond HIV/AIDS related forums for contributing to others, the men in this sample found many ways to give back to the world including small personal acts of kindness or charity, working on changing matters of social policy (e.g., discrimination complaints) and working on matters of global significance (e.g., environmental issues).

This category assumed significance in the lives of the men who were interviewed for two primary reasons. The first had to do with a recognition that working towards the betterment of themselves as a disenfranchised group was integral to their health and welfare. Secondly, it offered a supportive lifeline to a network of persons who could serve to validate them as people and legitimize and affirm their lifestyle. Among persons who did experience meaning in their lives, relationships and work (volunteer or paid) were offered as primary areas of meaningfulness.

DISCUSSION

This qualitative study has yielded some important information and phenomenological data on how the vast majority of HIV-infected individuals experience purpose, meaning and value in life following their diagnosis. However, given the sample size of 20, a general caveat should be noted: any quantitative results should be viewed as general trends or tendencies rather than interpreted as conclusions of any greater specificity.

Two primary phenomena were found to significantly influence the experience of meaning for the seropositive men as they confronted their illness. The most important of these phenomena was a sense of connection to or accountability towards some person or presence other than oneself. Over the course of the interviews the importance of this inter-connectedness with another was underscored time and again. The term inter-connectedness rather than interpersonal has been chosen because it is a more inclusive term which incorporates two types of association which were mentioned in addition to the association with other persons: the connection with a spiritual entity and connection with pets.

The second most important challenge these seropositive men faced was a shift or redefinition in their meaning, purpose and value in life. As the individual is diagnosed with HIV infection and the disease progresses, so often those aspects of life which once fulfilled a sense of meaning or purpose are lost (relationships [deaths of close friends or ex-partners to AIDS] or jobs or careers). Opening new channels for the expression and experience of life became instrumental in turning around an eroding sense of purpose for many of these men. Common examples of this were the discovery of new creative outlets for the expression of their feelings. For example, painting, journaling, writing short stories, poetry, film projects and participation in volunteerism (often with AIDS-related projects) offered new avenues of meaning and value for numbers of men who had to let go of old ones.

Employment and career involvement generally decreased or ended altogether for persons as they become symptomatic. This change in HIV status, coupled with the fact that occupation is considered a primary source of personal value for males in this culture, points to the importance of establishing other sources of personal worth, value, and meaning to assist seropositive persons in their adjustment out of the work setting.

For example, the importance of aesthetic involvement and artistic expressions which was found for a vast majority of the participants suggest ways to encourage seropositive persons to explore new modes of personal fulfillment, when old ones are no longer able to be sustained.

Beyond the richness and satisfaction and meaning experienced through relationships with others (including pets), social isolation studies confirm the impact of relationships on an immunological level as well with loneliness shown to affect natural killer cell (NK) activity in normal as well as clinical populations (Kiecolt-Glaser, Garner, Speicher, C., Penn, G. M., Holiday, J. E. & Glaser, R., 1984; Kiecolt-Glaser, Ricker, D., Messick, G., Speicher, C. E., Garner, W. & Glaser, R., 1984).

The absence of or struggle for a spiritual connection which affected over half of the men surveyed, offers fertile ground for religious leaders willing to transcend homophobic practices and doctrines. Given the need and desire for development in the area of spirituality for HIV-infected individuals, pastoral counseling programs that facilitate spiritual growth in a spirit of inclusivity could be in high demand among this disenfranchised segment of the population. However, mainstream religions would have to make significant changes in their own beliefs and values before these individuals could see their ministry as something other than hypocrisy and condescension.

By identifying primary ways in which seropositive persons experience a sense of meaning, purpose and value, and by discovering how this changes during the course of their illness, more insight to caregivers and health care professionals alike can be brought to bear on the process of easing the transition for persons just beginning the process.

REFERENCES

Batchelor, W. F. (1984). Psychological emergency. *American Psychologist*, *39*(11), 1279-1284.

Girogi, A. (1989). Some theoretical and practical issues regarding the psychological phenomenological method. *Saybrook Review*, *7*(2), 71-85.

Inhelder, B. & Piaget, J. (1958). *The growth of logical thinking from childhood to adolescence*. New York: Basic Books.

Joseph, J., Emmons, C., Kessler, C., O'Brian, K., Hacker, W., & Schaefer, C. (1984). Coping with the threat of AIDS: An approach to psychological assessment. *American Psychologist, 39,* 1297-1302.

Kiecolt-Glaser, J. K., Garner, W., Speicher, C., Penn, G. M., Holliday, J. E. & Glaser, R. (1984). Psychosocial modifiers of immunocompetence in medical students. *Psychosomatic Medicine, 46,* 7-14.

Kubler-Ross, E. (1969). *On death and dying.* London: MacMillan.

Lofland, J. & Lofland, L. (1984). *Analyzing social settings: a guide to qualitative observation and analysis.* Belmont, CA: Wadsworth Publishing Co.

Malyon, A. K. (1984). The psychological impact of AIDS on gay men. *American Psychologist, 39*(11), 1288-1293.

Marzuk, P. M., Tierney, H., Tardiff, K., Gross, E. M., Morgan, E. G., Hsu, M., & Mann, J. J. (1988). Increased risk of suicide in persons with AIDS. *Journal of the American Medical Association, 259*(9), 1333-1337.

Morin, S. G., & Batchelor, W. F. (1984). Responding to the psychological crisis of AIDS. *Public Health Reports, 99*(1), 4-9.

Nichols, S.E. (1984). Psychiatric aspects of AIDS. *Psychosomatics, 24*(12), 1083-1089.

Padilla, R. V. (1989). *Hyperqual Software and Users Guide Version 2.0,* Chandler, Arizona: Published by the author.

Ross, M. W., Tebble, W. E. M., & Viliunus, D. (1989). Staging of reactions to AIDS virus infection in asymptomatic homosexual men. *Journal of Psychology and Human Sexuality, 2*(1), 93-104.

APPENDIX

Meaning, Purpose and Value Questions

The following is a series of questions concerning how you experience(d) meaning and purpose in life since being diagnosed with HIV disease. I am interested in hearing both positive and negative ways that these areas of your life may or may not cover areas which are important to you. I want to encourage you to bring up aspects of your experience you are interested in which may go beyond these general questions.

1. Do you presently experience a sense of meaning, purpose or value in your life?
   a. If so, through what means?
2. Has this changed for you since being diagnosed HIV positive?
3. If this has changed for you, what or who has contributed to these changes?

4. I will describe six major categories through which people report experiencing a sense of meaning, purpose or value in their lives. With each one I would like you to comment on if it also holds meaning for you or if you have experienced struggles to find meaning, purpose and value through these areas since you have been diagnosed with HIV:

   a. Relationships (i.e., closeness to others, raising children).

   b. Self discovery (i.e., self-growth, learning about self).

   c. Spiritual fulfillment (i.e., developing a connection with one's higher self or higher power, however that be defined based on one's belief system).

   d. Acquiring knowledge (i.e., mastering skills, gathering new information).

   e. Aesthetic appreciation (i.e., arts, nature).

   f. Contributing to others or society (i.e., altruism, making a positive impact through work, contributing to scientific understanding of AIDS through participation in research).

5. Are there other areas of your life not described in these general categories which you feel have or currently provide you with a sense of meaning, purpose or value? If so, please describe.

6. How do you feel one's sense of meaning, purpose or value in life is affected being seropositive?

7. Has your general outlook on life or philosophy toward life changed since becoming HIV positive? Please describe.

8. At this point, I would like to give you a couple of minutes to think of anything else which is important to you regarding the content of this interview or anything else it has brought to your mind, giving your final comments to this interview.

Women and HIV

Willeke Bezemer, PhD

SUMMARY. Most of the scientific literature on HIV prevention campaigns (and medical and psychosocial health care) neglect the fact that women can be infected by HIV. This neglect is demonstrated in several ways: women are described as infectors and not as infectees, the typical disease profile in women is not described, and female sexuality and the position of women in society are not taken into account in prevention campaigns. The relative number of women infected with HIV rises. Research on women and HIV is needed to slow the rise in infection rates and adequately address the medical and psychological health care of HIV-infected women.

INTRODUCTION

Women are vulnerable to the human immunodeficiency virus (HIV) and are now contracting the disease at a faster rate than men. However, they are still under-represented among AIDS cases in Europe and the USA. In the Netherlands, 7% of all AIDS patients are women (NCAB, 1991). In England the incidence is 3% and in the United States it is 8.6% (totals approximately 60, 50 and 7000 respectively) (Jones and Catalan, 1989). Yet, AIDS has become the leading cause of death for women aged between 20 and 40 years, who live in major cities in the Americas, Western Europe, and sub-Saharan Africa (Chin, 1989). However, scientific studies, statistical reports, funding and media attention still lag behind when dealing with 'Women and AIDS/HIV.'

Address for Reprints: Dr. Willeke Bezemer, Langegracht 16, AH Maarssen, Holland 3601.

31

WOMEN AS INFECTEES
AND CARE OF INFECTED WOMEN

Looking at the care available to HIV infected women, prevention programs, test practices, scientific publications and media coverage, far more attention is being paid to women being infectors than to women being infectees. For example, there is a great deal of focus on the infected prostitutes who might infect their customers and much less attention is given to concerns about protecting the prostitute from the potentially infected customer. And, in the discussions about mandatory testing of pregnant women, the fear of transmission prevails over the care of women.

One of the main objections from feminist quarters is that most HIV projects being financed are aimed at helping white males (Patton, 1988). This is reflected in the well-developed medical and psychosocial care of infected homosexual men in Western European countries, while the amount of care of infected women is poorly developed. The Rutgers Foundation in the Netherlands has attempted to address this problem by establishing group counseling of seropositive women. The topics of these groups are related to women's lives and women's sexuality, and to the different disease-profile of women compared to men which is rarely mentioned in the medical literature.

TRANSMISSION IN WOMEN

In women, half of the cases of HIV infection still result from intravenous drug use. Heterosexual contact is the next most common means of transmission and is gaining (Whipple, 1991). Recent publications stress the (hetero)sexual conduct as the transmission way in IV drug users rather than the drug use itself (Ross, 1991; Verster, 1991).

In the USA, for example, the sexual way of transmission has increased considerably especially in women over the past three years: from 11% of all cases to 30% now (Guinan and Hardy, 1987; Campbell, 1990). By comparison, only 2% of the male AIDS patients in the USA were infected heterosexually.

Until recently, male-to-female-transmission and female-to-male-transmission were considered equally. Since the VI International Conference on AIDS in San Francisco (1990) it has been estimated that male-to-female transmission is five times as common as female-to-male transmission (Blans, 1990).

It has been hypothesized that penile-vaginal contact with an infected partner will infect a woman sooner than it does a man, because the infected semen tends to stay in the vagina for a while. Menstruation, gynecological infections, the usage of oral contraceptives and the use of an intra uterine device (IUD) also increase susceptibility to the virus (Piot et al., 1987; Kienzo, 1989). Piot and colleagues stress the growing susceptibility to HIV infection in women using oral contraception, possibly caused by alterations in cell-mediated immunity. The use of IUDs is a potential risk of (dangerous) pelvic infection, which may increase the pool of target lymphocytes in the vagina, thus increasing the susceptibility of HIV.

A European study group (1989) investigated the specific risk factors inherent in male-to-female transmission of HIV. Nine health centers in six European countries participated in the project which identified three important risk factors: a history of sexually transmitted disease in the preceding five years, a partner with fully developed AIDS and the practice of anal unprotected intercourse.

In addition to these physiological factors, there are also factors of a social character that may play a role in the increased risk of HIV infection among women. In Europe and in the USA, far more men than women are infected, so heterosexual women are to a much greater extent than are heterosexual men subject to the risk of meeting an infected partner. When a married male partner also has homosexual contacts, the possibility of his having sexual contacts with infected homosexual or bisexual men is not unthinkable. Most married men would never reveal their homosexual contacts to their wives due to the homophobic attitude in society. Consequently their wives are rarely aware of the risks of infection.

HIV PREVENTION CAMPAIGNS AND WOMEN

Whereas HIV prevention campaigns in the Netherlands have been targeted at men who have sex with men, IV drug users, as well as the general population (Moerkerk, 1990), none has been exclusively focused on women.

Currently, 'safer sex' is emphasized in most HIV prevention campaigns. The use of condoms during vaginal and anal intercourse is explicitly stressed as well as including information about the risks involved in sexual techniques such as unprotected oro-genital contact and kissing.

Until recently, the 'safer sex' concept was equal to the use of contraceptives. This particular notion was adopted by the average heterosexual woman who had (and still has) most of the responsibility in contraception. The question whether and which contraceptive measures are compatible with precautions against HIV, and how this can be integrated into a new 'safer sex' concept, confuses women. This is all the more confusing because men are inclined to take women's responsibility for protection against pregnancy as well as protection against an infection with HIV for granted.

The Dutch family planning institute, the Rutgers Foundation, in line with the WHO, stresses a mutual responsibility between women and men and the importance of both contraception and protection against STD and HIV. However, advocating the use of condoms as both a protection against pregnancy and as a protection against HIV simply doesn't work. Given the number of unwanted pregnancies, it is self-evident that condoms are not being used. Research indicates that women find it difficult to accept the use of condoms for several reasons: too much orientation on intercourse, it makes them feel like prostitutes, and the objections of the partners. And, if women do not object to the use of condoms and their partners do, they need to be assertive. This might cause a problem because most women are not assertive in sexual matters. They are being dominated by men's sexual desires. But also the concepts of romance, love and trust in relationships are a trap for women who want to protect themselves against HIV, because these concepts contradict the use of condoms.

By focusing on the use of condoms in 'safer sex' campaigns, intercourse seems to be the social norm of 'real' sex.

However, in examining attitudes of intercourse from a feminist point of view, Weeds (1987) found that five in every ten women liked having sex without intercourse, two out of ten disliked having sex with a male partner without intercourse, and three out of ten expressed no strong opinions about intercourse. Vennis (1989) found similar findings in his study of 850 'normal' couples, while Holland et al. found this also being the case in a sample of young women between 16 and 21 (1990).

So, why do women have intercourse more often than they really want? In heterosexual relationships it is not only women's needs and wishes that play a role in determining if intercourse occurs or not. In a recent Dutch study among 'happy marriages,' the dominance pattern was investigated. The researchers found that the husbands had the final say in housekeeping, the upbringing of the children, his wife's job, finance and sex (Komter, 1985). Because of this imbalance of power, women often consent to have intercourse on their husbands' terms and are blamed for wanting sex without intercourse. Other studies focus on the continuum of mild persuasion, through varying degrees of force, to brute attacks that women endure from their boyfriends and husbands when they want sex (Heelen, 1989; Kelly, 1988) to enlighten this phenomenon.

CONCLUSION

Today's society is in all its aspects very much dominated by men. Medical and psychosocial health care are not an exception to that rule.

In HIV prevention campaigns, scientific literature and in the media coverage, HIV is considered to be a male problem, though women are contracting the HIV infection at a faster rate than men do. The imbalance of power between genders inhibits the development of HIV prevention programs for women.

A much stronger involvement of women in all aspects of HIV–research, literature, prevention campaigns and the media–is urgently needed.

REFERENCES

Beelen, J. (1989). *Van Verleiden tot verkrachten*, Dekker, Amsterdam.
Blans, J. (1990). Nieuws uit San Francisco. *AIDS-info, 57*.
Campbell, C.A. (1990). Women and AIDS. *Soc. Sci. Med., 30*, 407-415.
Chin, J. (1989). European Study Group. Risk factors for male to female transmission of HIV. *British Medical Journal, 298*, 411-418.

European Study Group (1989). Heterosexual transmission of the immunodeficiency virus: a seroepidemicological study, *Archives for dermatological research, 298*, 411-418.

Guinan, M. E., Hardy, A. (1987). The epidemiology of AIDS in women in the United States, 1981 through 1986. *Journal of the American Medical Association, 257*, 2039-2042.

Holland, J., Ramazanoglu, C., Scott, S., Sharpe, S., Thomson, R. (1990). Sex, gender and power: young women's sexuality in the shadow of AIDS. *Sociology of Health and Illness, 12*, 336-350.

Jones, L. & Catalan, J. (1989). Women and HIV disease. *British Journal of Hospital Medicine, 41*, 526-538.

Kelly, L. (1988). *Surviving sexual violence.* Cambridge, Polity Press.

Komter, A. (1985). *De macht van de vanzelfsprekendheid.* VUGA, Amsterdam.

Moerkerk, H. (1990). AIDS prevention strategies in European countries. In: *Promoting Safer Sex*, ed. M. Paalman, Swets en Zeitlinger.

Patton, C. (1988). AIDS: Lessons from the gay community. *Feminist review, 30*, 105-111.

Parent, A. (1989). *Onvoltooide vooruitgang.* Van Loghum Slaterus, Deventer.

Piot, P. (1987). Heterosexual transmission of HIV. *AIDS, 1*, 199-206.

Rickert, V.I., Jay, M. S., Gottlieb, A., & Bridges, C. (1989). Adolescents and AIDS: Females attitudes and behaviors toward condom purchase and use. *Journal of Adolescents Health Care, 10*, 313-316.

Rienzo, B. de (1989). Heterosexual transmission of the immunodeficiency virus: A seroepidemiological study. *Archives for Dermatological Research, 281*, 369-372.

Ross, M. (1991). Sexuality and its risks in injected drug users. *Xth World Congress of Sexology*, Amsterdam.

Valdiserri, R.O., Arena, V. C., Proctor D. et al. (1989). The relationship between women's attitudes about condoms and their use: Implications for condom promoting programs. *American Journal of Public Health, 79*, 499-501.

Vennix, P. (1989). *Seks en Sekse*, Oberon, Delft.

Verster, J. (1991). Paper communication. *AIDS Florence '91*, Utrecht.

Vrouwen en AIDS, NCAB, 1991.

Weeda, I. (1987). *Eigenzinnige Erotiek.* Nijgh en Van Ditmar, Amsterdam.

Whipple, B. (1991). Paper communication, *Xth World Congress for Sexology*, Amsterdam, Session Women's Issues.

Prevention
of Heterosexual Transmission of HIV:
Barriers for Women

Anke A. Ehrhardt, PhD
Sandra Yingling, MA
Rezi Zawadzki, MS
Maria Martinez-Ramirez, CSW, MPH

SUMMARY. Heterosexually active women are at risk for HIV infection, yet many women do not practice safer sex. Unlike contraceptive methods such as the birth control pill, the only currently recommended HIV prevention method–the condom–is not under women's control and requires interpersonal sexual negotiation. In any case, consistent condom use is rare among heterosexual adults.

In assessing the reasons behind this phenomenon, we conducted focus groups with 78 women, primarily Latinas and Black women from high HIV seroprevalence neighborhoods. We collected information about contraceptive history, perception of HIV infection risk, acceptability of condoms to women and their partners, sexual negotiations with partners, and women's ideas for the development of new methods of HIV prevention.

Anke A. Ehrhardt, Sandra Yingling, Rezi Zawadzki, and Maria Martinez-Ramirez are affiliated with the HIV Center for Clinical and Behavioral Studies, New York State Psychiatric Institute and Columbia University College of Physicians and Surgeons.

Address all correspondence and requests for reprints to: Anke A. Ehrhardt, Director, HIV Center for Clinical and Behavioral Studies, 722 West 168 Street, New York, NY 10032.

The authors would like to thank Helen Gasch, MPH, for facilitating several focus groups and giving valuable feedback, and Hamida Khakoo, MD, of Lincoln Hospital's Department of Obstetrics and Gynecology. They are also indebted to Patricia A. Warne, PhD, for her invaluable assistance in preparing this manuscript. This study was supported by grant number 5-P50-MH43520 from NIMH/NIDA to the HIV Center for Clinical and Behavioral Studies.

37

Our study findings suggest the following: HIV prevention messages for women must take into account many women's lack of basic knowledge about their own sexual functioning; education strategies must be tailored to women's changing childbearing status and duration of primary sexual relationships over the lifecycle; negotiating condom use often threatens intimacy of sexual relationships and makes male partners suspicious or angry.

HIV interventions for women must consist of sex education, including anatomy and physiology. Sexual negotiation skills must be taught and HIV prevention messages must address many women's desire for pregnancy. In addition, development of new HIV prevention strategies must focus on methods under women's control that are outside of negotiation with a male sex partner.

INTRODUCTION

HIV infection rates among women continue to accelerate. In the United States, as many as 80,000 women of childbearing age may be HIV-infected (Gwinn et al., 1991). Male to female infection through sexual contact reportedly accounts for 33% of all AIDS cases in U.S. women (Centers for Disease Control, 1991), although the possibility of heterosexual transmission to women who have used intravenous drugs has not been assessed. Nationally, Black women comprise 51% of the women's AIDS cases attributed to heterosexual transmission, and Latinas comprise 23%.

In the New York metropolitan area, a cumulative total of 4,640 AIDS cases among adult women have been reported (New York City Department of Health, 1991). Many of these women are categorized as having been infected through intravenous drug use even though they likely also had heterosexual contact with a person at risk. It is striking that 24% of the new AIDS cases reported in 1991 among women in New York City are attributed to "sex with men at risk" and that an additional 22% of new cases among women are in the category "Other," which includes women who died before a transmission risk interview could be conducted.

Strategies for preventing heterosexual transmission of the virus are urgently needed in areas with high HIV infection rates. Communities with high prevalence of drug use are also communities in which there is a shrinking pool of potential sex partners who have not been exposed to HIV. Thus, women living in such communities, even if they do not themselves engage in high risk behaviors such as intravenous drug use, are at "geographic" risk of HIV infection through contact with infected men.

Current strategies for preventing heterosexual transmission of HIV rely on the use of condoms. However, it is now well documented that condoms are rarely used with either frequency or consistency. Estimates of condom use in heterosexual encounters range from 14% for married couples (Mosher, 1990) to 41% "regular use during intercourse" in a sample of college women (DeBuono et al., 1990). Approximately 46% of young Black and Latina women have their first experiences of sexual intercourse without any contraceptive or sexually transmitted disease prevention method (Forrest and Singh, 1990). Although 42% of a sample of young Black men reported using condoms at first intercourse, 49% reported using no (or ineffective) contraceptive methods (Sonenstein, Pleck and Ku, 1989).

Overall, between 1982 and 1988, women's reliance on their partners' use of condoms increased only slightly, from 12% of all contracepting women to 15% (Mosher, 1990). It is clear that women's protection against HIV is currently confounded by many long-standing issues of control over pregnancy and childbearing. Stein (1990) notes that the most effective measures of pregnancy prevention have been those that women control; she cites several studies indicating limited acceptability of condoms in heterosexual populations and has called for development of new HIV prevention methods that are within women's control. According to Ehrhardt (1988), reliance on condom use, which is ultimately controlled by the male partner, for the prevention of HIV transmission diminishes the control over their sexuality that women had gained with the availability of contraceptive methods that are independent of men (e.g., the pill, the IUD, and the diaphragm). Finally, women who are economically dependent on a male partner are rarely in a position to insist on condom use and thus cannot ensure their protection against HIV.

The purpose of our current investigation is to examine from women's perspective the barriers to protection against heterosexual HIV transmission; these include women's perception of their risk of HIV infection, women's report of acceptability of condoms, and women's negotiations with their sex partners. Women were also asked to imagine new HIV prevention methods they would consider ideal. We examined women's contraceptive history, including attitudes towards birth control and experience with various methods, which may be a major determinant of acceptability of HIV preventive methods. Overall, our goal is to collect information from women on which to base (a) more realistic interventions that will help women negotiate safer sex and (b) recommendations for development of new HIV preventive methods.

METHODS

Women between the ages of 19 and 45 years were recruited in a variety of settings to participate in discussion groups about contraception and HIV prevention methods. Participants were paid an average of $15 to complete questionnaires and to give their opinions in one-time focus groups averaging 90 minutes in duration. In the questionnaires, participants were asked for basic demographic data, including a description of ethnicity and level of acculturation. Ethnicity was assessed by asking participants about their ethnic self-identification and about their place of birth and that of their parents. The designation "Latina" in this sample describes women who identified themselves as Puerto Rican, Dominican, Cuban, Equa-dorean, Colombian, or simply Hispanic. The designation "Black" describes women who identified themselves as African-American, Negro, African, or Black.

The women also completed a contraceptive history form designed to compare current and past use of all contraceptive methods and an HIV knowledge questionnaire titled "Which Is Safer" (Koopman et al., 1990) that assessed their understanding of the relative risks of different types of sexual behaviors. Both forms were completed before participation in a focus group and provided baseline data prior to the group discussion.

Focus groups are part of a qualitative methodology designed not to provide information based on representative or random samples, but rather to investigate the range of possible responses and attitudes as well as group norms that may be found in a given setting (cf., Morgan, 1988). This approach can precede and complement more traditional survey techniques by uncovering areas not identified through structured survey methods.

The focus groups were conducted by two to three female facilitators (Latina, Black and White non-Hispanic), using a facilitator guide that listed topics to be covered. Focus groups began with a discussion of contraceptive methods that the participants had tried. A discussion of negotiating with sex partners about contraception was followed by questions about risk, including pregnancy, sexually transmitted disease, and HIV risks. Various forms of contraceptives, including contraceptive film (which forms a chemical barrier around the cervix) and the female condom (which is not yet on the market) were available for participants' inspection. The female condom, or pouch, has been described elsewhere (Drew et al., 1990); it is a polyurethane pouch to be worn intravaginally, and it may be as effective as the male condom in preventing sexual transmission of HIV. Finally, women were asked to imagine an ideal method for preventing sexual transmission of HIV. Participants were debriefed following focus groups, and given information on referral sources for a range of concerns including HIV counseling. Discussions were audiotaped for later transcription; all groups were conducted in English.

Content analysis of focus group transcripts involved two investigators separately reviewing transcripts to extract quotations within the key topic areas identified by the facilitator guide and subsequently developing categories based on responses within these topic areas. Categories not common to both investigators were discussed and those transcripts were re-examined jointly, often resulting in categories that may have initially been named differently being either subsumed under one name or remaining as distinct categories.

RESULTS

Description of Sample

A total of 78 women participated in eleven focus groups. The sample was not recruited based on risk factors such as a history of sexually transmitted disease or drug use. Rather, women were recruited within geographic locations, such as Harlem and the South Bronx, having high reported HIV seroprevalence. Sites included the street, women's health clinics, a family health fair, and a community college. Due to differences in recruitment strategies, more of the Latina focus group participants were community college students and hospital workers, whereas more of the Black focus group participants were patients in clinic settings and passersby on the street.

Of the 78 women who participated in focus groups, 35 were Latina and 41 were Black. Additionally, two women, one Caucasian non-Hispanic and one Asian, each participated in a focus group, but quantitative information from these two women is not included in this report for reasons of confidentiality. Demographic information as well as information on AIDS knowledge and contraceptive history is provided on most of the Latina and Black participants. The few women for whom we do not have complete data do not differ systematically from the overall sample.

These Latina and Black participants were similar in terms of age, years of education, and marital status (see Table 1), except that more Black women identified themselves as being in a common-law marriage than did Latinas, and more Latinas reported being divorced or separated than did Black women. About one quarter in each group had no children.

Quantitative Data

Of the remaining 76 Black and Latina women participating in focus groups, 71 (33 Latina and 38 Black women) completed forms that asked questions designed to assess knowledge of AIDS sexual risk behaviors and current and past contraceptive method use.

AIDS Knowledge

Based on a brief questionnaire (Koopman et al., 1990), we found that focus group participants had a good grasp of basic information regarding sexual transmission of HIV (Table 2). This 8-item HIV knowledge test asked women to choose which of two activities is the safer in terms of likelihood of HIV transmission. The test includes questions about various forms of casual contact and unpro-

Table 1. Demographic Information on Latina and Black Women.

	Latina Women	Black Women
	(N=33)	(N=38)
Mean age (years)	29.4	30.2
No children (percent)	24	24
	(N=31)	(N=38)
Mean education (years)	13.2	12.5
	(N=31)	(N=36)
Marital status (percent):		
Single (never married)	47	47
Currently married	28	25
Divorced/separated	22	17
Common-law marriage	3	11
	(N=31)	(N=37)
Work status (percent):		
Working full- or part-time	47	51
Currently not working	25	22
Educational forms of		
public assistance	22	3
Public assistance/welfare	6	24

tected sexual contact. Mean scores were 6.8 correct out of 8 questions for Latinas and 6.7 for Black women. Despite problems with both vocabulary and literacy, overall scores for participants in the eleven groups averaged 6.8 out of 8 correct (85%).

Current Use of Contraceptives

Prior to each focus group, participants completed a form about current and past contraceptive use. Participants could indicate more than one method concurrently in use or more than one reason they were not contracepting.

Of the 71 respondents, 26 (37%) reported they were currently using no form of birth control. Eight of the 26 reported they were not currently sexually active. Additional reasons for not using birth control included attempting pregnancy (10), currently pregnant (5), known fertility problems (3), religious prohibitions against birth

Table 2. Results of AIDS Knowledge Questionnaire, "Which Is Safer?",
for Latina (N=33) and Black Women (N=38).

"Which is safer...?" (percent correct)	Latina Women	Black Women
Giving blood, or receiving transfusion	94	90
Working in an office with someone who has AIDS, or contact with virus through open cut	97	97
Heterosexual vaginal intercourse with a woman who has AIDS, or anal intercourse with a man who has AIDS	67	76
Using a needle just used by a person with HIV, or a kiss on the lips with someone who has AIDS	97	97
A woman having unprotected vaginal intercourse with a man who has AIDS, or a man having unprotected vaginal intercourse with a woman who has AIDS	76	58
Having sexual intercourse with a person who shoots drugs, or spending time in the same house or room with a person who has AIDS	100	92
Homosexual anal intercourse with someone who has AIDS, or receiving a blood transfusion	88	87
Unprotected sexual intercouse with a lesbian, or unprotected sexual intercourse with a bisexual man	64	74

control (3), recent birth (1), and opposition by male partner of any form of birth control (1).

A variety of methods of birth control were reported currently in use (Table 3), the most common being the condom. Of the 10 Latinas stating that condoms were currently used, four reported their partners used condoms for each intercourse. Of 14 Black women, seven said their partners used condoms for each intercourse. Thus, of the 71 women surveyed, only eleven (15%) reported consistent condom use.

Following the condom, the most common contraceptive method was the birth control pill. The contraceptive sponge, spermicides, and penile withdrawal before ejaculation were reported currently in use both by Latinas and, to a somewhat larger extent, by Black women. Black participants also reported current use of contraceptive suppositories, the rhythm method, and diaphragms, whereas none of these methods was cited by Latinas.

Nine women reported surgical sterilization of themselves or their partner, mostly tubal ligation or hysterectomy of the woman, with two Latinas reporting vasectomy of their current male partner.

Current contraceptive use is notable in terms of HIV prevention for a number of reasons. First, these data suggest that, among women in the 30-year-old age range, it is likely that a sizable percentage (in this sample, 16 out of 71, or 23%) will either be attempting pregnancy, be currently pregnant, or have just delivered a baby. HIV prevention methods that interfere with conception therefore may not be acceptable to a significant number of women. Second, for women not currently seeking pregnancy, the type of contraceptive method they use gives us insight into the acceptability of HIV prevention methods that have contraceptive properties (i.e., condoms and spermicide). As shown in Table 3, 11 women in the sample reported current consistent condom use, and four reported current use of spermicides. These methods are used by fewer women than birth control pills (15 women) and tubal ligation or hysterectomy (seven women), both highly effective contraceptive measures that are coitus-independent and invisible, suggesting that these characteristics may be attractive in an HIV preventive method. Finally and disturbingly, some Black respondents reported reliance on ineffective contraceptive measures such as penile withdrawal before ejaculation, douching, vaginal suppositories, and the rhythm method. Clearly women who are attempting to prevent pregnancy by these methods lack the information and/or the means to implement effective contraception. This may be directly linked to traditional health beliefs among Black women, such as those described by Flaskerud and Rush (1989).

History of Contraceptive Use

Women reported no longer using some devices and methods that they had tried in the past; IUDs, diaphragms, sponge and douching were discontinued by many women. Condoms, birth control pills,

Table 3. Current Contraceptive Use in Latina (N=33) and Black Women (N=38)

| | Latina Women | | Black Women | |
	N	Percent	N	Percent
Any contraceptive method	20	61	25	66
Condom	10	30	14	37
Consistency of use*				
Each Intercourse	*4*	*12*	*7*	*18*
Most of the time	*4*	*12*	*4*	*11*
Rarely	*0*	*0*	*3*	*8*
Birth control pill	8	24	7	18
Surgical sterilization	5	15	4	11
Self (tubal ligation/hysterectomy)	*3*	*9*	*4*	*11*
Male partner (vasectomy)	*2*	*6*	*0*	*0*
Penile withdrawal	1	3	4	11
Spermicide	1	3	3	8
Contraceptive sponge	1	3	3	8
Douching	0	0	3	8
Suppositories	0	0	3	8
Rhythm method	0	0	2	5
Diaphragm	0	0	1	3

*Missing data on 2 Latinas.

and spermicides were the most commonly tried contraceptive methods for both Latinas and Black women and remained the most commonly used to date.

The contraceptive history profile of the 71 women providing information is depicted in Table 4. Three reported never having used any method of birth control. The method most commonly ever tried was the condom followed by birth control pills, spermicides, the rhythm method, and penile withdrawal before ejaculation.

The intrauterine device (IUD), diaphragm, and sponge had been tried by a larger percentage of Latina than Black participants. Also, herbal preparations and vaginal contraceptive film had been tried by Latinas but not by Black participants. More Black participants (N = 8) than Latinas (N = 4) reported having had an abortion.

From these data and those shown in Table 3, it is clear that

Table 4. History of Contraceptive Use In Latina (N=33) and Black (N=38) Women

| | Latina Women | | Black Women | |
	N	Percent	N	Percent
Any contraceptive method ever	31	94	37	97
Condom	22	67	25	66
Birth control pill	19	58	25	66
Spermicide	9	27	11	29
Rhythm method	9	27	11	29
Penile withdrawal	9	27	9	24
Intrauterine device	9	27	6	16
Diaphragm	8	24	6	16
Contraceptive sponge	7	21	4	11
Douching	6	18	8	21
Suppositories	4	12	4	11
Contraceptive film	1	3	0	0
Herbal preparations	3	9	0	0
Cervical cap	1	3	2	5

women in our sample have tried and discontinued a wide variety of birth control methods. For instance, more Latinas than Black women had ever used IUDs, diaphragms, herbal preparations and vaginal contraceptive film, but no Latinas reported current use of any of these methods. This variety may indicate women's willingness to look for a method with which they feel comfortable and which is effective.

QUALITATIVE DATA

These data are from all 78 women who participated in the focus groups.

Themes Identified in Focus Groups:
I. Barriers to Protecting Against HIV Infection

Women's opinions about contraceptive methods were solicited in focus groups; these data provide a deeper understanding of the quantitative information derived from self-administered questionnaires. Group discussions of contraceptive history provided a forum in which to discuss sexual negotiation in relation to male sex partners and also gave valuable information about the desirability of pregnancy. Since, as will be described below, many women did not perceive themselves to be at risk for HIV infection, family planning topics created a bridge to discussions of issues relevant to HIV risk such as fidelity, trust, and decision-making about sex partners.

Barriers to women's protection against HIV transmission in heterosexual intercourse include the perceived lack of HIV infection risk, especially among women in long-term or committed relationships, the low acceptability of condoms among men and women, and women's difficulties in sexual negotiations with their sex partners.

A. Detecting Personal Risk: Denial, Faith, the Personal Interview, and Evaluating the Odds

The first step in employing protection against sexual transmission of HIV is to perceive oneself to be personally at risk for infection. Some women never make a personal risk assessment, because they want to put the whole matter out of their thoughts (". . . *as far as I'm concerned, I like to be in control of what happens to me at all times, and it's very shaky; I try to just avoid thinking about the whole [HIV] situation altogether. I don't even think about it.*"). Other women feel too demoralized and overwhelmed by other circumstances in their life to determine whether they are at risk for infection ("*A lot of women don't care if they're protected or not . . . All the time she [sic] have experience with other diseases and a lot of vaginal infection and they don't care. And a lot of people in this country feel depression, and very poor people, they don't care.*").

Trust and faith play a key role in preventing women from making risk assessments. Religious faith and belief in the institution of marriage can lead to a feeling that one is exempt from risk ("*I've been married for many years to my husband . . . I know him pretty well and we also have the fear of God in our life. And I know if I do something I'm accountable to God, so maybe that makes us a little different. I've never thought of getting AIDS from him.*").

Women in long-term relationships may feel able to assess a partner's fidelity–and serostatus–by knowing his routine and schedule; the perception of exclusivity of affection and friendship can preclude even considering a partner's history (*"I've been with my husband eleven years, but he's never given me no signs of anything outside. I have no friends . . . Everything is the family, the children and me."*).

For some women, the apparent trust they place in their partner carries with it an implicit threat of retribution should the partner prove unfaithful and infectious: *"He ain't never given me no reason for me to think that he's doing anything and I'm not giving him no reason. You know, he goes to work and then comes from work. We talked about [HIV] but as far as I'm concerned if I was to ever get it, it would be from him . . . and I'd kill him. I'd wait til he goes to sleep, tie him up, cut off his penis and I'd just slash him up."* Also, a woman's trust in a partner's fidelity can be linked to her perception of *his* infection fears: *"I don't think my husband would sleep around because he's terrified of AIDS. He's really afraid. He's convulsive over the whole thing . . . he will spray Windex on his hands to get his hands clean. And he thinks the Windex is going to kill the AIDS virus if he's got any . . . So I know that he will not sleep around unless he's desperate or crazy. He knows I'll kill him–or the AIDS will kill him."*

Suspiciousness about HIV status may go hand-in-hand with detecting what are considered signs of infidelity, bad judgment, or lack of sexual control. Women may feel comfortable rejecting men with these characteristics and may assume that this screening has left them with a pool of HIV-negative partners to choose from (*"When you encounter people that, you know, just do it for the hell of it, you know their hormones are not in check. Then you have to give that a second thought . . . So basically you have to go on a little bit of everything–character and how this person presents himself to you and everything else."*). This approach is consonant with public health messages urging an interview of a prospective sexual partner as an effective screening strategy.

Elaborate attempts to develop personalized ways of assessing HIV risk within a relationship are not uncommon. In fact, many women develop their own sense of personal risk in a kind of at-home social scientist approach. One woman describes the method she used to arrive at the conclusion she and her partner are at low risk for infection; note that her assessment is based on measuring odds of infection per number of partners, and also on her partner's truthfulness:

> *I've sat down with him and I've asked him what kind of relationships he'd had before he and I got together. I wanted to know more or less what kind of sexual habits he had before we got together. I don't particularly care for a man who's been with Tom, Dick and Harriet and then all of a sudden it's me, because you never know what could have happened between Tom, Dick and Harriet, as they say. To this day every now and then we talk and we still think about what the possibilities are . . . we've sat down and we've said, if it came down to the nitty-gritty what kind of risk, on a scale of one to ten, where would you put yourself? And, I scored myself very low. I said zero to one, really, because I'm sexually active . . . but it's always been with a specific partner. It's now like my son's father is one man and I'm with my next husband, and in between I may have had like two relationships . . . And I asked him about his relationships and I asked him to do the same thing, and he's more or less the same as I am. Whether or not I believe him is up to me, because all men are going to sugarcoat whatever it is that they want to sugarcoat and they will downplay whatever it is they want to downplay . . . And they say if you bring up the same conversation more than once within different periods of time, if the same answer appears that means it's really from the heart and it's the truth, but if they start changing it a little, you're going to think twice about it and then you're going to get a little stronger with the questions that you are asking . . .*

For many participants in the focus group setting, discussion of HIV risk was not personalized because they felt they were not at risk; for example, they felt they were in mutually monogamous relationships. Discussions of HIV risk in the group were often elicited by asking "What should women in general do?" or "If your situation changed, how would you protect yourself *if you were at risk?"*

B. When are Condoms Used–or Not: Watching for Symptoms, Preventing Pregnancy, Condoms as Punishment, Aesthetics, Testing the Relationship

It is remarkable that condom use is often framed as something women can do. Our focus group participants commonly used phrases such as "I tried to use them." Women develop strategies for keeping the perception of risk at bay, including frequent visits to the doctor: *"I think for us that don't use condoms, we have to use our better judgment as to the type of people we are, and yes, we do take a risk, but this is the choice that we take because we don't want to use those condoms. And basically how we keep ourself [sic] well, I go to the doctor every six months. My gynecologist is right around the corner. I have regular Pap smear tests, anything that needs to be done. If anything hurts my body area, I'm like a doctor myself, I go away with a prognosis. And that's what I do. I keep myself clean and hope for the best."*

For a woman to be protected against heterosexual transmission of HIV requires interpersonal negotiation and often direct confrontation. Women's negotiations with their partners about condom use may go most smoothly when no other contraceptive is in use; pregnancy prevention may be more compelling and immediate than HIV prevention: *"We have been using condoms and we never forget them and we're real careful. First of all, because I'm not using birth control and I don't want to become pregnant. And secondly because with the HIV virus, it scares the shit out of me so I just don't want to take any chances. I use mostly the excuse that I don't want any kids."*

Women's trust in condoms may need to be enhanced, since breakage is a common fear: *"I tried condoms–mentally I couldn't do it. I wasn't sure about the safety and pregnancy and the whole thing, especially when they break after you finish."*

Consistency of condom use varies. Some women find it easier to introduce condom use as a punishment after they suspect a partner of infidelity: *". . . my husband [says] 'No!' but I make him use it because . . . because you never know when . . . men are men. That's mostly why I use the condom. I mean, I don't use it all the time, but there's sometimes that I say, 'Use it.' Because you never know . . . But I feel uncomfortable for some reason if he was out for a long time or . . . I mean, you're supposed to have trust, I understand that . . . I usually try to make him use it, but there's times when he doesn't want to, and that's the times when [problem comes in].*" Disturbingly, condoms are sometimes seen as a method which male partners can be persuaded to use only after a woman has a visible indicator of a vaginal infection: "*I'm scared of infections, diseases, whatever. So the slightest little thing and he has to wear a condom or we're not doing anything . . . If I don't have a discharge, then we'll just be bare . . . I don't use any birth control because I want a baby now. I want to get pregnant.*"

Partner refusal to wear condoms was widely reported; the wife of a recent immigrant reported that her husband said, "'*No, I'm not a schoolboy . . . and if you don't trust me, I'll go back to Africa where you trust me and I feel comfortable.' He don't like using condoms.*" Armed with education, women have confronted men on the issue, and tested their relationships: "*[I went to] a conference on AIDS . . . I talked to my boyfriend and explained about that. He said, if you want I use condom, I going to separate with you. And I separate from him.*"

When condoms are tried, it is with varying degrees of discomfort, and women continue to educate ("*I'm not saying in general, but men could be a little ignorant, and it's like women are known for yeast infections . . . So you have to explain these things, that this comes from there. Here, read up on this, give him a pamphlet. You have to let them know how this thing works and how your body works*"), to negotiate ("*One of my first questions was whether or not he was willing to use condoms 'cause I don't really want to use birth control. I'd rather my partner take care of it, make sure they're responsible. And, well, . . . I found this guy and he was willing and he's willing to be responsible*") and to confront ("*Some of the [men] will come up and say, 'I'm too big to wear a condom.' I say, 'How big can you be?'*").

Aesthetically, condom use leaves much to be desired. Women report giving up the method as too uncomfortable, perhaps because lubricants are not used in conjunction with condoms ("*I explained to him the use of the condom. He tried to use it but with the condom I don't feel good because I think there's something rough inside . . . That's why I don't use anything*"). Condoms are seen as a threat to sexual pleasure ("*[he] doesn't really complain. I don't know, when you come, I guess it don't feel as good in a condom as it would if the condom wasn't there . . .*"), and this can lead to discarding the method ("*[Without condoms] I feel good and I can tell he feels good. I just don't want to drive him away*").

Women who determine themselves to be at risk for infection may choose not to have sex: "*I got what I want, and that's my daughter. [I've been abstinent for seven years] while the disease is going around.*" Many women reported that since condoms are the only HIV-preventive available, they had no choice but to rely on condoms: "*to me, the safest one is the condom. As uncomfortable as it is, it is the only thing.*" Although most women who reported condom use on their survey forms did not indicate separate use of spermicides, many had heard the message that some spermicides have virucidal properties: "*condoms and spermicide . . . make sure it has nonoxynol-9.*"

Although none of the focus group participants indicated she knew she was seropositive, many women reported the effects of failure of their partners to use condoms in terms of a different outcome: pregnancy. "*I got off the pill and I had told my husband–you know, we started to get involved–and I told him to use the condom so I don't get pregnant. He says, 'I don't know, I don't know. You won't get pregnant, you won't get pregnant.' And I said 'Use it!' and I'm fighting with him while were 'doing it.' Well, anyway, I had the baby.*"

For some women with personal knowledge of AIDS, proof of a partner's seronegativity is something worth fighting for. One focus group participant knew that her husband had had sex with a woman whose relatives had died of AIDS; she insisted on proof of her husband's seronegative status, and stayed in the relationship: "*. . . she came to my home and took my husband . . . I go to the hospital and I say I'm the [wife] let me see the [HIV test] record. I don't sleep with him if I don't see the record.*" Knowing someone with AIDS can create skepticism about traditional methods of coping:

"There's another friend of mine who was a Jehovah's Witness, and her husband was using drugs and she died . . . so this is something that prayer, forget a prayer, I want the condom . . . So I don't care if you're with him every day. You ain't with that man every day. And not to say he's using drugs. You don't know if he's all that faithful. That shit is real, and there's no cure."

Themes Identified in Focus Groups:
II. Imagining an Ideal Method of HIV Prevention

A. Detection

Initially, rather than describing a barrier device for preventing HIV transmission, focus group participants were interested in ways to insure detection of a man's infected status prior to intercourse. One idea was an automatic, on-site blood test (*"like they have the glucose here, you can test for sugar and stuff, if they had a test for [HIV], something that you can stick your finger, let me see the blood and it tests negative, 'OK, let's go, we're ready'"*) and another idea involved a virus-detecting condom (*"an HIV detector . . . a type of condom that they put on them and it changes color and it tells you whether they have anything"*).

B. Reactions to the Female Condom

Many focus group participants had never seen a sample of a vaginal pouch, or female condom, before the focus group. Many felt positively towards the idea of a barrier method for women which prevented HIV transmission: *"I guess if you're having sex with different partners or whatever, I think it is a good idea for the woman to protect herself . . . I think this is a good idea because it lets you be in control."* Often, even though they had been told that the female condom was only for demonstration purposes, women asked after a focus group if they could take the female condom home (*"I probably would try it."*).

However, many women expressed reservations about a condom to be worn by women. They had strong reactions to its size (*"When they make a smaller one, get in touch with me.''*), designed to cover the vaginal walls: *"condoms for women. That's the weirdest thing I've ever seen. It looks like an elephant trunk.''* The female condom's visibility was of concern (*"I think having this on your outer lips makes you look a little funny.''*), and it also raised gynecological concerns among women who had had problems with diaphragm use: *"I could see some women using it, but I wouldn't because of my experience with the diaphragm. It was very painful"* or women who felt uncomfortable with vaginally inserting devices: *"Besides a penis, I don't like the idea of sticking nothing else up there. I'm serious. Diaphragms, nothing . . . I stuck a tampon up in me and it felt funny . . . When they came up with all these methods, I was like, you know, 'How can people have sex with these things sitting up in them?' I just can't.''* or women who felt uncertain about their own anatomy: *"I would be afraid of this [female condom] going in . . . I don't know what would be the outcome of it.''*

Women did not like the female condom because, like various barrier methods of contraception, it can interfere with sexual spontaneity and sensation: *"I don't know about anybody else, but I like to get petted and touched and stuff like that, and doing this, inserting it beforehand, means that you will of course have to prepare for the whole thing . . . .''* Some women were concerned that they would have to use different HIV-preventive methods for different sexual practices: *". . . and the other issue is: it's all right for vaginal intercourse, but what about anal intercourse?''*

The issue of negotiating with one's sex partner, which is a problem with condoms for men, continues with the female condom: *"Personally I don't think men would be really thrilled about this. I know that most of the time they like to touch, they like to feel, they don't want plastic around.''* Women were concerned that men would be suspicious of a woman's motivation for wearing a female condom: *"I think that if I were to use it and not inform the person that I was wearing something like this, and they all of a sudden saw one of these . . . you know, 'You got something I don't know about?''* This theme was a fairly common reaction, involving suspiciousness about women's genitalia: *"But when the men touch you, feel something, . . . 'What do you have in there?''* The detectability of the female condom raised fears that the intimacy of the relationship would be broken by the specter of disease: *"I guess it would start something in the relationship of 'now you don't trust me.'"*

C. Ideal HIV Methods: Characteristics of Existing Birth Control Methods

Some women felt that the burden of contraception had too long been women's responsibility and sought an HIV prevention method, for example a pill to be taken orally, like the birth control pill, that men could use (*"something like a birth control pill for men. Something for men for a change, not the woman all the time. Because the woman always has to go through the PMS, the menstrual period, everything. Men shouldn't have it so easy"*). However, other women indicated that this could pose a problem involving trust that the partner was in fact using an HIV preventive method (*"I'd rather have something that I would definitely do than to take a chance that maybe they are [lying] . . . Something that you see, have a pill that he can take right there in front of you and you say 'OK, I'm protected.' And that would be OK; but if it's something like 'I did it last night' or 'I used it this morning. . .'*). In fact, this line of inquiry produced a good deal of hostile responses about women's desires for men to experience the physical discomforts women do (*"I want the whole thing to go to them–the pregnant thing, the period bit, everything"*) or just to have men experience pain (*"needles. I want them to have pain . . . right in there [penis] for all I care."*).

In terms of developing methods of HIV prevention for women to use, some indicated that using an intravaginal device would be preferable (*"I would design it for the woman, being inserted into the vagina, and removing it like once a month when you have your periods. And just keep it in there. That would be great."*). However, others expressed reservations about methods which remain in the vagina, including women who reported unpleasant experiences with intrauterine devices.

Women's experiences with spermicides are particularly important in light of efforts to develop virucides against HIV. Many reported spermicidal foam made them feel unpleasant or unclean: "*It dissolves . . . so then you have all this gooey stuff coming out . . . he ejaculates, so you have more gooey stuff coming, so you just got one big total mess.*" Some participants had positive reactions to c-film (vaginal contraceptive film), because it would not be "drippy and messy" like foam, and would like to see a virucidal film developed. Even though women had reservations about long-term effects of birth control pills, many said they would use an HIV-preventive pill if it were available, even with some familiar side-effects: "*pills [like birth control pills] . . . I'd rather gain weight than to know I have AIDS . . . I'd rather gain 1000 pounds.*"

Many women would like to see an inoculation against HIV, given at the same time as routine inoculations against, for example, rubella, or similar to subdermal hormonal contraceptives: "*If they're going to model something after birth control, they might consider this Norplant thing to protect you all the time.*"). However, for others, it is considered unpleasant and unsafe to use needles ("*no injection. The needle might be dirty.*") or break the skin ("*I don't want nothing under my skin.*"). One woman fantasized about a technique involving immersion: "*I was just thinking about this movie 'Cocoon,' where they went into the water. If both the male and the female were to make love in the water, then they'd be like protected from everything.*"

In sum, many women felt that an ideal HIV prevention method, if used by women should not be visible, but if used by a man should be obvious. The ideal method would be coitus-independent, could not be felt during intercourse, and would not have systemic side-effects.

Themes Identified in Focus Groups:
III. Differences Among Latinas and Black Women

All focus groups were conducted in English. Marin (1989) estimates that only 15% of Hispanics nationally prefer to speak in English and an additional 60% are proficient in English, although they prefer to speak Spanish. Thus, the Latinas in our focus groups are not representative of the 25% of Hispanics in the United States who do not speak any English.

We did not find issues or themes that were of concern exclusively for Latinas or exclusively for Black women in our sample. Cessation of some currently available contraceptive methods did differ by ethnicity, with Black women more frequently discontinuing birth control pills, citing hypertension as a side-effect, and Latinas more frequently mentioning side-effects from their attempts to use IUDs.

Black women in our sample tended to have more children on average (mean = 3.3) than the Latinas in our sample (mean = 2.3) and were more likely to be in a long-term relationship outside marriage, i.e., "common-law marriage" (11% vs. 3%). These demographics reflect population characteristics for urban minority women.

In negotiating contraceptive method use, Latinas in our sample more frequently mentioned having relied on covert means to achieve their goals (*"So what I did was I went and had an IUD put in. And he never knew the difference. Never. Until I took it out five years later to get pregnant. And to this day, he still doesn't know that I had that IUD put on."*), whereas Black women more often related direct confrontations about contraception (*"when I was going to the Nation of Islam [religious group], this guy wanted me to use the rhythm method . . . you wasn't supposed to take no birth controls . . . He didn't like condoms, you know how they are. So we did have a lot of disagreements . . . so after a while I did win because he wasn't getting none unless he did what I said."*).

Latinas and Black women told similar stories of domestic violence. A Latina related: *"[my cousin] got pregnant, and I guess he didn't want the baby, and he let her know the hard way. He went and threw her down the stairs . . . and I said, 'Next time you hurt my cousin like that, you're the one who's gonna go out the window, not down the stairs.'"* A Black woman reported: *"I didn't know a lot of things about AIDS and HIV and that stuff. I just thought maybe . . . he would get AIDS and I would get it so I just like, that's it . . . I'm staying in a shelter . . . and now he still tries to contact me, he calls. About a month ago he wrapped an extension cord around my neck and tried to choke me while I was carrying my son . . . Now he's real scary and I'm a little afraid of him. And if he finds out I'm going with somebody now he would probably try to kill me."*

In terms of HIV prevention, the idea that having a single sex partner makes for "safe sex" is a common one. A Black woman in our sample said, *"I'm going to get the [HIV] test very soon because I'm about ready to get married now. I never wanted to marry anyone, but I said, 'I better get married; it's too dangerous out here.' And he's [been] in love with me for years now. So I don't think he would give me AIDS."* And a Latina, who is also concerned about taking precautions against HIV, said, *"My partner and I just met, and this disease is around and you have to use protection. If you've been with your partner for a while, then it's different . . . I don't think I would use anything if we were together [for a while]."*

DISCUSSION

Current HIV prevention messages emphasize abstinence, monogamy, reduction in the number of sex partners, interviewing partners for sexual histories, and the use of condoms. These messages do not address many issues salient to heterosexually active women. Even though the vast majority of women with HIV infection are between the ages of 20 and 45, few HIV prevention programs target women "of reproductive age," who are generally perceived to be loyally monogamous and thus not at risk (Carovano, 1991). This study has identified several issues that must be addressed if HIV prevention programs for women at risk for heterosexual transmission are to succeed.

Perception of Risk

Our focus group participants, women from high HIV-seroprevalence communities, have a relatively high degree of AIDS knowledge and a keen awareness of the HIV threat in their midst; but, many do not feel that they personally are at risk for HIV infection. This perception is particularly strong among women in long-term or "committed" relationships and may influence a woman's motivation to protect herself, especially by negotiating condom use. We were struck by the persistence and ingenuity of many women who acted as at-home social scientists, developing their own yardsticks for risk assessment. Some women seem to remain in a protracted assessment period because attempting to negotiate condom use is too difficult, and the process of assessing risk may persevere as a way of denying that a woman should implement prevention behaviors. Those women who are in committed, long-term relationships (including marriages) often did not assess themselves to be at risk for contracting the virus based on the assumption that they and their male sex partner are currently mutually monogamous. The emotional experience of being in a close, trusting, and faithful relationship was seen by many as completely antithetical to discussing or employing HIV prevention methods.

Thus, we conclude that, even armed with appropriate knowledge of HIV transmission routes and relative risks of sexual acts, women may not see themselves as personally at risk for HIV infection via their male sex partner. This can have deadly consequences, as seen in a study of women attending an inner-city Baltimore prenatal clinic. Although 40% of women who were found to be seropositive reported intravenous drug use, another 47% denied risk factors for HIV infection (Barbacci et al., 1990). The authors conclude that sexual transmission was the probable explanation and that the women were apparently unaware of the risk status of their sexual partners. In a study of Hispanic women who were homeless, intravenous drug users, or the sex partners of intravenous drug users, the majority interviewed did not report the threat of AIDS as a common fear. The authors ascribed this to the women's need to focus on economic survival, but also noted the contribution of cultural factors, such as many Latinas' proscriptions against discussing sexual practices openly (Nyamathi and Vasquez, 1989). Finally, our observed denial of personal risk mirrors the results of a pilot study of non-Hispanic white women in Rhode Island (Zierler, Newman, and Cheung, in press), many of whom saw pregnancy as an immediate problem, and sexually transmitted diseases as a remote and invisible problem.

HIV infection does not provide any warning signs, and this is of great concern. Women reported to us that condom use often comes into play after a woman has developed a yeast infection or some other gynecological manifestation. This stance parallels women's attitudes toward treatable sexually transmitted diseases, but it can lead to deadly consequences: partners of unknown serostatus can infect their monogamous female partners with an untreatable and fatal virus long before symptoms are visible. There is evidence from other studies that women who have altered their sexual behavior in the direction of risk reduction are those who have been treated for a sexually transmitted disease (Cochran and Peplau, unpublished).

Desire for Pregnancy

Adult women who are heterosexually active also experience a conflict between protection against HIV and the desire for pregnancy. Almost one quarter of our focus group participants were attempting pregnancy, pregnant, or immediately postpartum at the time of interview and reported using no birth control or sexually-transmitted disease prevention method. The role of motherhood is at odds with current state-of-the-art HIV prevention, as noted by Worth (1989); and women in long-term relationships may be more willing to set guidelines about the types of sex in which they will engage (e.g., refusing anal intercourse) than about condom use, which would preclude the possibility of pregnancy. For many women, their reproductive role defines their personal identity (Carovano, 1991). Therefore, the development of HIV prevention methods that do not have contraceptive properties should be a priority, allowing women to choose disease protection without giving up reproductive options.

Existing Methods for Prevention of Heterosexual Transmission

Our study offers several insights into the problems with existing methods of HIV prevention and the characteristics that novel methods should possess. The major existing method is the male condom. Condoms present crucial problems of gender and power negotiation to the woman who tries to introduce them into her sexual relationship. HIV prevention in the context of heterosexual sex reflects the ongoing difficulties women have in negotiating with men and protecting themselves from accidental pregnancy and from sexually transmitted diseases. With HIV prevention, however, issues of trust and fears of alienating the male partner come to the forefront, especially for those women in committed or (assumed) monogamous relationships. For some women, broaching the subject of disease transmission and condom use is an insurmountable barrier. A smaller subgroup approached the question with pragmatism and recommended to their regular partners that condoms be used if the partners had additional female sex partners.

In general, however, negotiation with a male sex partner to encourage condom use requires that a woman go against many culturally defined sexual scripts and concepts of acceptable masculine and feminine gender roles. Some women alluded to trying to negotiate condom use during the act of intercourse; others noted that the threat of domestic violence and monitoring by some men of their wives' whereabouts already creates a tense climate between men and women.

Socioeconomic factors can play an enormous role in contraception and HIV prevention. Within the Black community especially, women are reported to have lost power in their relationships with men even as men's economic standing has declined (Fullilove et al., 1990), thus widening a gender-based difference seen in other heterosexual settings. In the United States, the relative frequency of unplanned and unwanted births is consistently higher among women of lower socioeconomic status than among higher status women (Jones et al., 1988), perhaps reflecting the inability of the former to negotiate contraception with their sex partners. These same barriers can be expected to operate in negotiations around HIV prevention.

The second barrier to condom use is its lack of aesthetic appeal to women. This objection applied as well to the female condom, or vaginal pouch. Some women did not like the idea of inserting a device into their vaginas. Other concerns were similar to those for the male condom: it interrupts sexual activity, it may reduce sensation, it may break. However, some participants were intrigued and wished to try the pouch.

Lack of aesthetic appeal applies as well to the other recommended HIV preventive–spermicides. Along with a reluctance to insert anything (e.g., an applicator) into the vagina, some women did not like the "messiness" and viscosity of spermicidal foams, although they knew that nonoxynol-9 has virucidal properties. These issues may be addressed by appropriate education.

Ideal Methods for Prevention of Heterosexual Transmission

A range of opinions about ideal methods of HIV prevention were identified, many of which indicated that methods employed by women should not be visible, so that negotiation is limited. Conversely, women wanted methods employed by men to be visible, so that a woman might know that the method is being used.

Ideas about ideal method of HIV prevention mirrored women's experiences with existing birth control methods: skepticism about safe placement of any HIV barrier methods was rooted in subjects' experiences with unplanned pregnancies due to barrier method failure; and suspicion about systemic effects and teratogenicity of any inoculation or injection seemed related to known side-effects of birth control pills. However, women were interested in the development of coitus-independent methods of HIV prevention that would have a systemic effect.

While some women were comfortable with an injection, others were fearful of needles. While some women wanted a device that could be worn intravaginally for extended periods of time, some were fearful of developing infections from prolonged contact with the device and others were uncomfortable with vaginal insertion regardless of duration. Previous exposure to a range of contraceptive devices had created very definite and fixed opinions about the types of methods they would be willing to try. The female condom, because of its visibility, was rejected by some women, but others felt that it would be a useful barrier method against HIV that women could use if they discussed the method with partners prior to intercourse. Development of a spermicide with virucidal properties was of interest to some women, but only if it did not have the properties of currently available spermicides, which are often described as "messy" and as making women feel unclean.

Education as Part of a Prevention Program

Our focus groups raised many issues indicating that adequate education about HIV risk, sexual anatomy and physiology, method utilization, and negotiation skills will be crucial to the development of effective methods of preventing heterosexual transmission of HIV.

Although AIDS knowledge was fairly high in this sample, there is still some confusion between blood transfusions and blood donation and some opinion that anal sex is risky among heterosexuals but vaginal sex is not. Some women were surprised to learn from others in their focus group that engaging in oral sex may carry a risk of HIV infection. As mentioned earlier, perception of self at risk may be important in establishing motivation to use a prevention method.

Focus group participants' discussions of their experiences with a large range of contraceptive methods indicated that method failure resulting in pregnancy is not uncommon. Women are willing to try methods of birth control, but monitoring a woman's introduction to a new method is crucial to the continuation of use. There are lessons for HIV prevention in this information. Teaching women about their own genitalia and the range of physiological changes related to maturation, the menstrual cycle, childbirth, and so forth is a necessary component in successful utilization of contraceptive methods and thus of methods for HIV prevention. Vaginal insertion of any device can pose problems for women who do not receive adequate anatomical and utilization information: one of the focus group participants tried to use tampons when she was a virgin, experienced pain, and has never used them since. It may take only one bad experience, be it a woman's discomfort, her male partner's discomfort, or various aesthetic considerations of method, for a contraceptive method to be discontinued. Other studies of adult heterosexually active women have shown that discontinuation of birth control methods is common (Grady, Hayward and Florey, 1988); in one sample of married women who were not attempting pregnancy, a chosen birth control method was abandoned within the initial year of use by 28% of the sample. Spermicides, diaphragms, and condoms were the most frequently abandoned methods.

In developing HIV prevention strategies for heterosexual women, education and intervention components must be tailored to the life cycle issues of women (Ehrhardt and Wasserheit, in press). These include issues around preparing for menstruation, sexual initiation, birth control method, options in childbearing, body changes during and after pregnancy, and HIV prevention during menopause. Similarly, a woman's life circumstances must be taken into consideration; different styles of intervention may be appropriate for women with a single male partner or multiple partners, a woman who is in committed or casual relationships.

For all women, regardless of life cycle issues, the development of an HIV preventive method that women can use, which is outside of negotiations with male sex partners, is an urgent and pressing need.

CONCLUSIONS

In developing strategies for HIV education among heterosexually active adult women, women's life circumstances need to be evaluated and educational efforts tailored to women's changing status in relation to childbearing and longevity of primary sexual relationship. Women in long-term and "committed" or assumed mutually monogamous relationships need to know that they may be at risk for HIV infection, especially if they live in geographically "at risk" neighborhoods.

Condom use in preventing HIV infection requires that women negotiate with their male sex partners. The impact of such negotiations, including the potential for loss of culturally-determined social status, domestic violence, or even economic disadvantage, must be addressed. Educational interventions must take into consideration women's value systems, including ethnically-specific values (Marin, 1989). They should also include a question that weighs HIV risk against other risks in a woman's daily life: "What impact would negotiating condom use have on this woman's life circumstances?"

HIV interventions for women must include sex education, including anatomy and physiology; sexual negotiation not specific to HIV issues must be taught; and HIV prevention messages must address many women's desire for pregnancy.

Development of new HIV-prevention strategies must focus on methods that women can control outside of negotiation with a male sex partner. Recommendations for the future may include marketing currently available spermicides having virucidal properties as virucides to be used by women whether or not their male sex partner agrees to condom use.

REFERENCES

Barbacci, M.B., Dalabetta, G.A., Repke, J.T., Talbot, B.L., Charache, P., Polk, F., and Chaisson, R.E. (1990). Human immunodeficiency virus infection in women attending an inner-city prenatal clinic: ineffectiveness of targeted screening. Sexually Transmitted Diseases, 17, 3, 122-126.

Carovano, K. (1991). More than mothers and whores: Redefining the AIDS prevention needs of women. International Journal of Health Services, 21, 1, 131-142.

Centers for Disease Control (1991). HIV/AIDS Surveillance Report: U.S. AIDS cases reported through March 1991.

Cochran, S.D., and Peplau, L.A. (unpublished). Sexual risk reduction behaviors among young heterosexual adults. Submitted for publication.

DeBuono, B.A., Zinner, S.H., Daamen, M., and McCormack, W.M. (1990). Sexual behavior of college women in 1975, 1986, and 1989. The New England Journal of Medicine, 322, 12, 821-825.

Drew, W.L., Blair, M., Miner, R.C., Conant, M. (1990). Evaluation of the virus permeability of a new condom for women. Sexually Transmitted Diseases, 17, 2, 110-112.

Ehrhardt, A.A. (1988). Preventing and treating AIDS: the expertise of the behavioral sciences. Bulletin of the New York Academy of Medicine, 64, 6, 513-519.

Ehrhardt, A.A. and Wasserheit, J.N. (in press). Age, gender and sexual risk behaviors for sexually transmitted diseases in the United States. In: Research Issues in Human Behavior and Sexually Transmitted Diseases in the AIDS Era, J.N. Wasserheit, S.O. Aral and K.K. Holmes. American Society of Microbiology, Washington, D.C.

Flaskerud, J.H. and Rush, C.E. (1989). AIDS and traditional health beliefs and practices of black women. Nursing Research, 38, 4, 210-215.

Forrest, J.D. and Singh, S. (1990). The sexual and reproductive behavior of American women, 1982-1988. Family Planning Perspectives, 22, 5, 206-214.

Fullilove, M.T., Fullilove, R.E., Haynes, K., and Gross, S. (1990). Black women and AIDS prevention: a view towards understanding the gender rules. The Journal of Sex Research, 27, 1, 47-64.

Grady, W.R., Hayward, M.D., and Florey, F.A. (1988). Contraceptive discontinuation among married women in the United States. Studies in Family Planning, 19, 227.

Gwinn, M., Pappaioanou, M., George, J.R., Hannon, W.H., Wasser, S.C., Redus,

M.A., Hoff, R., Grady, G.F., Willoughby, A., Novello, A.C., Petersen, L.R., Dondero, T.J., and Curran, J.W. (1991). Prevalence of HIV infection in child-bearing women in the United States. Journal of the American Medical Association, 265, 13, 1704-1708.

Jones, E.F., Forrest, J.D., Henshaw, S.K., Silverman, J., and Torres, A. (1988). Unintended pregnancy, contraceptive practice and family planning services in developed countries. Family Planning Perspectives, 20, 2, 53-67.

Koopman, C., Rotheram-Borus, M.J., Henderson, R., Bradley, J.S., and Hunter, J. (1990). Assessment of knowledge of AIDS and beliefs about AIDS prevention among adolescents. AIDS Education and Prevention 2, 1, 58-70.

Marin, G. (1989). AIDS prevention among Hispanics: needs, risk behaviors, and cultural values. Public Health Reports, 104, 5, 411-415.

Morgan, D.L. (1988). Focus Groups As Qualitative Research. Qualitative Research Methods Series 16. Sage Publications, Inc.: Newbury Park, California.

Mosher, W.D. (1990). Contraceptive practice in the United States, 1948-1988. Family Planning Perspectives, 22, 5, 198-205.

New York City Department of Health AIDS Surveillance Unit (1991). AIDS Surveillance Update, First Quarter, 1991.

Nyamathi, A. and Vasquez, R. (1989). Impact of poverty, homelessness, and drugs on Hispanic women at risk for HIV infection. Hispanic Journal of the Behavioral Sciences, 11, 4, 299-314.

Sonenstein, F.L., Pleck, J.H. and Ku, L.C. (1989). Sexual activity, condom use and AIDS awareness among adolescent males. Family Planning Perspectives, 21, 4, 152-158.

Stein, Z.A. (1990). HIV prevention: the need for methods women can use. American Journal of Public Health, 80, 460-462.

Worth, D. (1989). Sexual decision-making and AIDS: why condom promotion among vulnerable women is likely to fail. Studies in Family Planning, 20, 6, 297-307.

Zierler, S., Newman, L.F., and Cheung, D. (in press). Epidemiological and ethnographic methods for research in high risk behavior. In: Research Issues in Human Behavior and Sexually Transmitted Diseases in the AIDS Era. Ed. J. N. Wasserheit, S.O. Aral, K. K. Holmes. American Society for Microbiology, Washington, D.C.

Denial as a Barrier for HIV Prevention Within the General Population

Theodorus G. M. Sandfort, PhD
Gertjan van Zessen, PhD (cand.)

SUMMARY. On an individual level, the accurate perception of the risk of HIV infection is a necessary condition for taking preventive measures in one's sexual behavior. This perception generally depends upon a variety of factors. Denial as one of these factors is the focus of a study carried out among a representative sample of 1001 Dutch citizens between the ages of 18 and 50 (mean age 32 years), who have been interviewed face to face. Scales have been developed to assess the tendency to reason away the risk of HIV infection and the tendency to play this risk down. The results of this study show that the tendency to deny the risk of HIV infection influences the way people deal with HIV/AIDS. People who sexually have been at risk and who reason this risk away don't acknowledge the fact that they have been at risk. These people also less often worried about the possibility of being infected. In general, the stronger the tendency to reason away the risk of infection, the less often subjects worried about their future risk of getting infected. People who play down the risk of infection are also less apt to take any precautionary actions in future sexual encounters. In the future planning of HIV prevention activities this tendency to deny the risk of HIV infection

Theodorus G. M. Sandfort is Co-Director of the AIDS Research program at the Department of Gay and Lesbian Studies, University of Utrecht. Gertjan van Zessen holds the same position at the Netherlands Institute for Social Sexological Research, Utrecht, Netherlands.

All correspondence should be directed to Theodorus G.M. Sandfort, Department of Gay and Lesbian Studies, University of Utrecht, P.O. Box 80.140, 3508 TC Utrecht, Netherlands.

The authors thank Ernest de Vroome for his assistance in analyzing the data and Lena Nilsson Schönnesson for her constructive comments. The study has been funded by the Netherlands Foundation for Preventive Medicine (28-1147) and The Dutch Ministry of Welfare, Health and Cultural Affairs (90.047).

69

should be acknowledged in order to improve efforts to reach their goals.

The statement that behavior change is the only medicine against HIV, even when a vaccine has been developed, has almost become a platitude. This does, however, not alter the validity of the statement. In the meantime, data from studies among gay men show that it is not only behavior change that is important. Gay men who have changed their behavior may not always continue to engage in safe behavior (Stall, Ekstrand, Pollack, McKusick & Coates, 1990), so activities directed at sustaining changed behavior are critical as well. However, empirical data about behavior change in the general population are scarcely available (Van Zessen & Sandfort, 1991).

Sexual behavior change, regardless of sexual preference, depends on a variety of factors, among others, attitudes and social norms (Fishbein & Middlestadt, 1989), and self-efficacy (Bandura, 1989). It is further important to keep in mind that safer sex behavior is not just accomplished by independent individuals, but that it comes about in an interaction in which two or more persons are involved (Salt, Boyle, & Ives, 1990).

From an individual perspective, attitudes and skills are irrelevant as long as a person does not consider himself to be at risk in terms of his or her sexual behavior. So, an accurate perception of the risk one runs is a necessary although not sufficient condition for taking preventive measures (Weinstein, 1989; Paalman & Sandfort, 1990).

The perception of the riskfullness of one's behavior generally depends upon a variety of factors, like denial, information and awareness of the issue (Weinstein, 1988) and attitudes towards sexuality (Byrne, 1983). We would like to suggest that the same factors apply to HIV related issues. If denial plays a role in the perception of risk of HIV transmission, it may seriously impede effective prevention. One consequence of denial may be that people seclude themselves from prevention messages. Another one may be that despite being aware of the risk of transmission, individuals do not apply this information to their own behavior.

Sexual behavior change is related to whether one knows people who are HIV infected or who have AIDS. As a consequence of personal confrontations with HIV/AIDS related issues, the awareness of potential risk might be heightened. However, these confrontations may also lead to an increased level of anxiety, and, consequently, to a stronger need to deny the potential danger.

Especially in the beginning of the pandemic, knowledge about HIV was related to behavior change (Becker & Joseph, 1988). As a consequence, it is quite likely that factors like knowledge and information are related to the perception of risk as well. Not knowing how the virus can be transmitted makes it impossible to make valid judgments about one's behavior.

As has been shown in several studies, people with permissive attitudes towards sexuality are more open for information about sexuality (Byrne, 1983). In the context of HIV this might imply that the more permissive attitudes one has towards sexuality, the bigger the chances that one has an accurate perception of one's potential risk of HIV infections.

This study focuses on denial as one of the factors that might influence the perception of one's risk to get infected with HIV. If it can be shown that denial plays a part in the perception of the risk of HIV transmission, this should have clear cut consequences for programming prevention policies. In studying the extent to which denial plays a role in the perception of one's sexual risk, the potential role of knowledge of HIV/AIDS, social proximity to HIV/AIDS and attitudes towards sexuality should also be taken into account.

The aim of this paper is threefold: First we will explore the possibility to assess denial as a factor influencing the perception of the risk of HIV infection within the general population. Two forms of denial are assumed to be operative: reasoning away the risk and minimizing or playing down this risk. A second aim is to explore whether subgroups can be identified as to the degree of denial of risk. Thirdly, we will explore the way in which denial might influence the process of adopting safer sex practices. Within this context, denial might influence the way AIDS is being experienced, the labeling of one's past sexual behavior, and future sexual behavior in terms of risk for HIV infection. It is expected that people who deny the risk of infection will perceive AIDS to be less threatening and will less often perceive themselves to be at risk, even when this is inconsistent with their actual or future behavior.

In studying denial of risk of HIV infection, it should be realized that risk itself is not randomly distributed among members of the general population. This might obscure the actual role of denial. To get a clearer view of the way denial influences the perception of one's past sexual behavior, we have focused on those who in the year preceding the interview had run some sexual risk of infection. With respect to future behavior, the potential role of denial was examined among those people for whom future risk was opportune. This means that they considered the possibility of having a new sex partner or thought it to be expedient to take precautions in the future. At the same time it should be clear that people cannot avoid potential risk by subscribing to certain attitudes. Whether one is at potential risk or not depends exclusively on one's sexual behavior and that of one's partner.

METHOD

Subjects

Data for this study were collected by means of personal interviews among a representative sample of 1001 Dutch citizens between the ages of 18 and 50 (Van Zessen & Sandfort, 1991). Of the participants 421 were male and 580 female. Mean scores and frequency distributions have been tested for gender differences. If these differences have been found they are mentioned in the text. Correlations between variables and multivariate analyses have not been computed separately for men and women.

The interviews were conducted in 1989 by trained male and female interviewers. The duration of the interviews averaged 75 minutes. The mean age of the participants was 32 years (sd: 8.94). The interviews took place in privacy in the subjects' homes.

Of those being interviewed, 73% were involved in a steady, monogamous relationship. Another 6% had a steady relationship but had, in the year preceding the interview, also had extra-relational sexual contacts with one or more persons. Nine percent had had sexual contacts in the preceding year, but were currently not involved in a steady relationship, and 12% had had no sexual contacts at all.

Instruments

The interview was predominantly structured with a fixed answering format. Some open questions were posed as well. Additionally, self-administered questionnaires and card sort tasks were used.

Denial of risk of HIV infection was measured by a pool of items, a priori categorized in two dimensions: reasoning the risk away (8 items) and playing down the risk (8 items). These items were included in a self-administered questionnaire.

Three aspects of *knowledge of HIV/AIDS* were assessed: knowledge in general (e.g., number of people having AIDS), ways of transmission of HIV, and ways in which transmission can be prevented. The questions probed for knowledge of accurate facts as well as for endorsement of certain misconceptions (e.g., transmission by using public toilets). The answers of 19 questions were combined in an HIV/AIDS knowledge score (alpha .75) by adding up the right answers and converting the resulting scores to a scale ranging from 0 to 100 (none to exclusively correct answers). The mean score was 58.9 (sd = 18.8; see Appendix A); there were no significant differences between men and women as to their knowledge about HIV and AIDS.

Social proximity of HIV/AIDS assessed the extent to which subjects have been confronted with HIV/AIDS related issues. A converted score on a dimension of 0 to 100 (none versus several, different confrontations with HIV related issues) based on answers to four related questions (alpha .62):

- whether one knew of someone in one's personal surroundings who has taken any measures in order to prevent HIV infection.
- whether one believed there were people within one's personal network who ran the risk of being HIV-positive or of becoming HIV-positive.
- whether one knew people who had tested for HIV.
- whether someone had ever personally known someone who has or had AIDS?

The mean HIV/AIDS proximity score was 25.8 (sd = 28.78); there were no significant gender differences.

To determine whether subjects had run any sexual risk of infection, their sexual behavior with steady and casual partners in the preceding year was assessed in detail. Participants were considered to have been at risk if they had had:

- unprotected intercourse (vaginal or anal) outside of a monogamous relationship and/or
- unprotected intercourse in a steady relationship in which the partner had had sex with a third person in the past year.

According to this definition, 15% of the men and 10% of the women had run some risk in the year preceding the interview (Sandfort, Van Zessen, Van Griensven, Straver & Tielman, 1991). This behavioral measure of risk should be distinguished from an absolute measure, in which information about infectivity and the prevalence of HIV has been taken into account as well.

Attitudes towards sexuality were measured on the dimension restrictiveness (1) and permissiveness (5) by using a Likert type scale with ten statements about sexuality and gender roles (alpha .78; mean score: 3.33, sd = .74; see Appendix B); there were no significant differences between men and women.

The extent to which subjects *worried about HIV/AIDS related issues* and certain topics in general was measured by means of a card sort task. By sorting out cards, participants had to indicate on a five point scale (never = 1; almost always = 5) to what degree they had been upset about a variety of general and personal matters during the past few months. The HIV related topics included: "That I am already infected with HIV" and "That I will get infected with HIV" (mean scores respectively: 1.17 and 1.93; no significant differences between men and women). The scores on topics not related to HIV were averaged to measure a person's general tendency to worry about things (alpha .72; mean score: 1.99, sd = .45; see Appendix C).

Subjects' *estimation of their future risk* to get infected with HIV was assessed in two consecutive steps. First the question was asked whether the participants thought that in the future they might get into a situation where the risk existed of becoming infected with HIV via sexual contact. To those respondents who did not rule this out completely, a second question was posed: "To what extent do you think you will run a risk of becoming infected with the virus in the future?'' Subjects could rate their chances on a scale comprising the following alternatives: ''very unlikely, quite possible, very likely, don't know/not sure.'' Taking the answering distribution into account, the answers to both questions are summarized in one score: future infection is completely ruled out (56%), is quite unlikely/don't know (34%), is quite possible/very likely (10%). Men ruled out future infection significantly less often than women did. This two step approach has been taken because it was expected that participants for whom future sexual risk actually should be excluded, would not be inclined to say ''none'' to prevent the unfavorable impression of being too decided.

RESULTS

A scale analysis of the denial statements produced two reliable scales measuring the extent to which people reason away the risk of HIV infection or play down this risk (alpha respectively .79 and .73; Table 1). A factor analysis produced almost the same results; for conceptual reasons the a priori grouping of items into subscales was preferred. The participants differed in the extent to which they reasoned away the risk of HIV infection or played down this risk. Mean scale scores were 2.26 (sd = .81) and 1.73 (sd = .62), respectively. Men and women did not differ in the tendency to deny risk. Both tendencies are related to each other: subjects who reasoned away the risk of HIV infection were also more inclined to play down this risk (r = .51, p < .00). However, since both tendencies showed different patterns of relations with other variables they are dealt with separately. There were only few relationships with the tendency to play down the risk of HIV infection; only significant relationships will be presented.

It is not possible to distinguish clear subgroups of people who do deny the risk of HIV infection. However, some trends can be observed, especially regarding the tendency to reason away the risk of infection. This reasoning away was done more often among those subjects who were older (r = .12, p < .00), had a lower degree of education (r = −.36, p < .00), came from lower social classes (r =

TABLE 1. Denial of the risk of HIV infection scales

	% (completely) agree	item rest correlation
REASONING AWAY THE RISK OF INFECTION *		
You only run the risk of becoming infected with HIV when you're a homosexual or when you inject drugs	24	.58
If you've never had a venereal disease, you probably can't get AIDS	7	.57
I won't get infected with HIV because that sort of thing never happens to me	26	.55
You run the risk of infection only when you have casual sexual partners	53	.50
If you wash yourself well after sexual contact, you run very little risk of infection	6	.46
I'm not the kind of person that that sort of thing happens to	28	.52
If you can trust the other person, then you don't have to do anything to prevent infection	20	.44
If you know someone a little, then you know right away if you run a risk	25	.40
PLAYING DOWN THE RISK OF INFECTION **		
In my opinion the enjoyment of sex and exercising caution just don't go together for me	18	.36
You should just enjoy sex even if you run some risk	8	.57
Taking risks with sex makes it extra exciting	6	.46
The chance that I'll be infected with the virus is so small that I accept the risk	25	.41
If you get infected, it's just hard luck	10	.38
The threat of AIDS is greatly exaggerated	7	.43
The chance of infection also makes sex more exciting	2	.49
You just have to accept the risk of infection	4	.49

* alpha is .79.
** alpha is .73.

−.26, p < .00), had a right wing political orientation (r = .11, p < .00), went to church more often (r = −.13, p < .00), and lived in smaller communities (r = −.11, p < .00). Multiple regression analysis (stepwise) showed that the variables age, education, social class and political orientation independently contributed to the explanation of the tendency to reason away the risk of infection (R = .39).

Additionally, there were group differences with respect to relationship status. Subjects who were involved in a steady, monogamous relationship and subjects who had had no sexual partners in the preceding year more often reasoned away the risk of HIV infection compared to those who had been single but sexually active or who had had extramarital partners (means respectively 2.31, 2.35, 1.94 and 1.89, F = 10.28, p < .00). This indicates that denial is related to relationship status and that it at least partially reflects the actual situation. It should, however, be noticed that infection cannot be prevented by placing oneself in a non-risk group. This erroneous tendency may be a negative side effect of the application of the concept of 'risk groups' in discussions about prevention.

The tendency to play down the risk of HIV infection was more equally distributed among the population. It was more often present among participants who had a lower degree of education (r = −.16, p < .00) and who came from lower social classes (r = −.21, p < .00). In a multiple regression equation only the last variable had predictive value.

The findings also indicate that denial of the risk of infection is related to attitudes towards sexuality, to knowledge of HIV/AIDS and to HIV/AIDS proximity. Subjects with permissive attitudes towards sexuality were less inclined to deny the risk (reasoning away r = −.42, playing down r = −.18, both p < .00). This suggests that people with permissive attitudes are not only more open for information about sexuality, but also for information about their potential risk of HIV infections.

Participants who displayed correct information about HIV/AIDS were more apt less often to deny the risk of infection (reasoning away: r = −.53, playing down: r = −.28, both p < .00). This suggests that denial might be a consequence of misinformation; however, by denying the danger of HIV/AIDS, people may also close themselves off from information about HIV/AIDS, resulting in less correct knowledge. In support with the latter interpretation is the relationship with HIV/AIDS proximity: subjects who did not deny the risk of infection reported more personal confrontations with HIV/AIDS related issues (reasoning away: r = −.37, playing down: r = −.17, both p < .00). Not having been confronted with people who got tested or who are HIV infected, HIV/AIDS might be such a distant and abstract issue that it is hard to imagine that one might personally be at risk. A dynamic interpretation is possible as well: denying the risk of infection might foster selective perception and guard someone from threatening confrontations with HIV/AIDS related issues. Probably both interpretations are valid at the same time.

Taken together in a multiple regression analysis, sexual attitudes, knowledge about HIV/AIDS and HIV/AIDS proximity were all independently related to denial of risk (reasoning away: R = .60; playing down: R = .30).

General Perception of AIDS

As suggested by the results, denial of the risk of HIV infection is related to the way in which people perceive AIDS. Denial also seems to be related to the participants' estimates of their relative risk. By asking to what extent they, compared to other Dutchmen of their own age, thought they ran a greater or smaller risk of becoming HIV infected, only 5% reported running greater risk. Twenty eight percent thought their risk of infection to be equal to that of people of their own age, and 68% reported to run a lower risk. Women reported more often than men that, compared to people of their own age, they ran a lower risk. On a group level, there should be a balance between the proportion of subjects who estimate their risk as relatively greater and relatively lower then others (Weinstein, 1980). This is clearly not the case. While on a personal level it is not possible to say who is underestimating the risk, on a group level underestimation is certainly present. This underestimation is positively related to reasoning away the risk of infection (r = .21, p < .00). The relation between denial and relative risk supports the validity of the interpretation of the denial scales.

At a first glance, there was no relation between denial and worries the subjects had about the possibility of already being HIV infected. However, such a relation was present when only participants who did not exclude the possibility of already being infected (N = 197) were considered. Within this group, persons who less strongly reasoned the risk away, more often worried about the possibility that they might already be infected (r = −.22, p < .00). It could be argued that this relationship could be explained by a general tendency of people to worry. However this correlation remains significant when controlled for this general tendency. Additionally, worries about being infected did not seem to be an effect of personal confrontations with HIV/AIDS related issues.

Denial was also related to the tendency to worry about future risk of infection; the stronger the tendency to reason away the risk of infection, the less often subjects worried about their future risk of getting infected (r = −.17, p < .00). These worries seem to be partially activated by the social proximity of HIV/AIDS (r = .20, p < .00). A multiple regression analysis showed, however, that reasoning away played an independent part as well. Both relationships with worries about past and future infection suggest that for people who do not deny the risk of infection, it is relatively more easy to experience negative feelings related to the possibility of being infected.

HIV/AIDS might not only be a personal threat. It may also be experienced as a threat to one's immediate social network and to society at large. Both threats were quite differently being experienced. Thirty-seven percent of the subjects did not experience HIV/AIDS as threatening to their social network, while 2% did not think HIV/AIDS to be threatening for society. Men and women do not differ in the extent to which they perceive HIV/AIDS to be threatening to their personal network; women, compared to men, perceive the threat of HIV/AIDS to society to be bigger.

Those subjects who played down the risk of infection perceived HIV/AIDS as less threatening to one's personal network and to the society at large (respectively r = −.10 and r = −.21, both p < .00). A multiple regression analysis showed that playing down only had an independent deadening influence on the threat of HIV/AIDS to society at large, and not on the threat of HIV/AIDS to one's personal network.

Subjects who experienced HIV/AIDS as threatening to their social network were less inclined to reason away the risk (r = −.18, p < .00; also significant when controlled for HIV/AIDS proximity). Reasoning away the risk was, however, not related to the perceived threat of HIV/AIDS to society. These findings suggest that the threat of HIV/AIDS to one's personal network elicits negative feelings, which some people feel inclined to suppress. Although HIV/AIDS is considered to be more threatening to the society at large, this threat seems to be more abstract. It might be that the negative feelings this more general threat elicits are not strong enough to induce some people to suppress them.

Sexual Risk in the Past

When asked to consider one's sexual behavior in the past, most subjects (80%) completely ruled out the risk of already being HIV infected. The female participants were more apt to do so then their male counterparts. One man and one woman in the sample stated that they were seropositive. Respondents who reasoned away the risk of infection more strongly were more inclined to rule out this possibility (r = −.23, p < .00). Combined in a multiple regression analysis with HIV/AIDS proximity, knowledge of HIV/AIDS, and attitudes towards sexuality, reasoning away did not have an independent influence on the risks people considered of being infected (R = .35).

It is of course possible that those who denied the risk of infection really did run no or less risk. Because detailed information about the subjects' past sexual behavior was collected, it was possible to check the subjects' own judgment about the safety of their behavior to a more objective measure. The participants' own judgment about the risk they had run and the objective risk measure correlated highly. However, of those who excluded the risk of infection, 8% had run some risk according to the objective measure. Of those subjects who thought that infection might have happened 71% had actually run some risk. This discrepancy occurs as often among men as among women.

To get a better understanding of the potential role of denial, only those subjects who objectively had been at risk for infection were considered. Within this group the same relationship between reasoning away the risk of infection and the subjects' personal judgment was identified. Participants who did not acknowledge their sexual behavior as risk-bearing showed, in contrast to those who did acknowledge the risk, a stronger tendency to reason away the risk (mean scores respectively: 2.18 and 1.76, $F = 8.15$, $p < .01$). Participants who did not acknowledge the fact that they had potentially been at risk for HIV infection more often than those who did acknowledge the risk agreed with statements like: "I won't get infected with HIV because that sort of thing never happens to me" and "I'm not the kind of person that sort of thing happens to."

Within the group of subjects who objectively had been at some risk, persons who more strongly reason away the risk of infection also less often reported that they had done something in the past to prevent HIV infections ($r = .25$, $p < .01$; for the total group: $r = .21$, $p < .00$).

Future Risk

Denial of the risk of infection also seemed to influence people's estimate of future sexual risk. The tendency to reason away the risk of infection was strongest among those subjects who excluded the possibility of getting into a situation where the risk of HIV transmission existed. Participants who thought it quite possible or even likely that they might get infected in the future seem to reason away the risk of infection less often ($r = -.21$, $p < .00$). These subjects more often agreed with statements like: "You only run the risk of becoming infected with HIV when you're a homosexual or when you inject drugs," "If you've never had a venereal disease, you probably can't get AIDS," and "You run the risk of infection only when you have casual sexual partners."

Perception of future risk was also related to knowledge of HIV/AIDS and HIV/AIDS proximity, indicating that people who were better informed about HIV/AIDS and who had been personally confronted with HIV/AIDS related issues, more often considered themselves to be at risk for future HIV infection by sexual contact. However, in a multiple regression analysis reasoning away the risk of infection had the strongest predictive value.

Does denial affect people's intention to do something to prevent HIV infections in future sexual encounters with a new partner? Because future risk is not equally likely for each subject in the population, only those who expected to have new sexual partners or who did not exclude possible situations in which they might get infected are being considered here (N = 627). Although a question about future prevention might induce socially desirable answers, 26% of the men and 14% of the women said that they would definitely not take any precautions or *might* do something to prevent infection. It is important to notice that the wording of the question about future prevention included the suggestion that one might be willing to accept some risk. Taking into account both types of denial, data showed that those subjects who played down the risk of infection were less inclined to take precautions (r = .30, p < .00). In a multiple regression analysis some other variables also predicted a negative intention. However they did not outshine the impact of playing down the risk of infection. Participants who were less intended to do something to prevent HIV infection more often agreed with statements like: "In my opinion, the enjoyment of sex and exercising caution just don't go together," "You should just enjoy sex even if you run some risk," and "If you get infected, it's just hard luck."

DISCUSSION

The results of this study show that the tendency to deny the risk of HIV infection influences the ways people deal with HIV/AIDS. People who sexually have been at risk and who reason away this risk don't acknowledge the fact that they have been at risk, and, probably as a consequence, they less often worry about possibly being infected. The same tendency is operative within the whole sample with respect to worries about being infected in the future. Denying seems to have a muting effect on the negative feelings resulting from the threat of HIV/AIDS for one's personal network and for society at large. People who play down the risk of infection are less apt to take any precautionary actions in future sexual encounters.

These results come from a cross sectional analysis. As a consequence, it is difficult to interpret the causality of the relationships. Does denial really serve the function of suppressing negative feelings, or does it serve other purposes? It would be helpful to have more insights in the way the mechanism of denial is operative. To get these, the use of qualitative measures might be indispensable.

To what extent does the tendency to deny the risk of infection threaten effective prevention? This question can be answered from an individual and from an epidemiological point of view. On an individual level, denial of risk might be fatal. The ways of calculating risks on a group level do not apply to the individual level. It is not possible to get a little bit infected, like it is impossible to get a little pregnant. From an epidemiological point of view, the seriousness of denial depends on the prevalence of HIV. It is quite obvious that within gay networks, denial will have a more devastating effect compared to networks of heterosexuals, at least when we look at Western countries.

The findings from this study have two clear implications for prevention. Realizing that denial is influencing the way people deal with the risk of infection, one of the preventive efforts should be directed at conquering this barrier. This could be done by making visible that HIV also affects people who do not belong to traditional risk groups. Another implication has to do with the general tone of HIV prevention campaigns. Without denying the seriousness of AIDS–an important motive to practice safer sex–these campaigns should not promote the tendency to deny the risk by increasing the anxiety for AIDS. In this way, people might seclude themselves from information which in some instances could save their lives.

REFERENCES

Bandura, A. (1989). Perceived self-efficacy in the exercise of control over AIDS infection. In Mays, V.M., Albee, G.W. and Schneider, S.F. (eds.) *Primary prevention of AIDS: Psychological approaches* (pp. 128-141). Newbury Park, CA: Sage.

Becker, M.H., & Joseph, J.G. (1988). AIDS and behavioral change to reduce risk: A review. *American Journal of Public Health, 78,* 394-410.

Byrne, D. (1983). The antecedents, correlates, and consequents of erotophobia-erotophilia. In Davis, C.M. (ed.) *Challenges in sexual research* (pp. 53-75). Syracuse: Society for the Scientific Study of Sex.

Fishbein, M., & Middlestadt, S.E. (1989). Using the theory of reasoned action as a framework for understanding and changing AIDS-related behaviors. In Mays, V.M., Albee, G.W. and Schneider, S.F. (eds.) *Primary prevention of AIDS: Psychological approaches* (pp. 93-110). Newbury Park, CA: Sage.

Paalman, M., & Sandfort, Th. (1990). Promoting safer sex among the public at large. In Paalman, M. (ed.) *Promoting safer sex* pp. 199-216. Amsterdam: Swets & Zeitlinger.

Salt, H., Boyle, M., & Ives, J. (1990). HIV prevention: current health promoting behaviour models for understanding psycho-social determinants of condom use. *AIDS Care, 2,* 69-75.

Sandfort, Th., Van Zessen, G., Van Griensven, G., Straver, C., & Tielman, R. (1991). *Risk-bearing behavior and risk awareness in three distinct samples of the Dutch population.* Paper presented at the VII International Conference on AIDS (M.D. 4084). Florence 16-21 June 1991.

Stall, R., Ekstrand, M., Pollack, L., McKusick, L., & Coates, T.J. (1990). Relapse from safer sex: the next challenge for AIDS prevention efforts. *Journal of Acquired Immune Deficiency Syndromes, 3,* 1181-1187.

Van Zessen, G., & Sandfort, Th. (1991). *Seksualiteit in Nederland. Seksueel gedrag, risico en preventie van AIDS.* Amsterdam: Swets & Zeitlinger.

Weinstein, N.D. (1980). Unrealistic optimism about future life events. *Journal of Personality and Social Psychology, 39,* 806-820.

Weinstein, N.D. (1988). The precaution adoption process. *Health Psychology, 7,* 355-396.

Weinstein, N.D. (1989). Perception of personal susceptibility to harm. In Mays, V.M., Albee, G.W. and Schneider, S.F. (eds.) *Primary prevention of AIDS: Psychological approaches* (pp. 142-167). Newbury Park, CA: Sage.

APPENDIX A. HIV/AIDS related knowledge scale *

	correct answer	% correct answers	item rest correlation
You can tell when someone's infected with the virus	(completely) agree; neutral	16	.33
If you're infected with the virus, it can take years before you become sick	(completely) disagree; neutral	34	.24
By drinking out of a glass from someone who has AIDS	totally impossible	54	.44
By shaking hands with someone who has AIDS	totally impossible	77	.43
By a mosquito bite or other blood-sucking insect	totally impossible	34	.27
Through sexual intercourse	quite possible	91	.23
By kissing someone who has AIDS	virtually impossible; totally impossible; don't know	82	.26
Through vaccination in a Dutch hospital	totally impossible	27	.24
Through anal sexual contact	quite possible	83	.17
From a pregnant woman to her baby	quite possible	80	.25
Through drawing blood for a transfusion	totally impossible	18	.25
By using public toilets	totally impossible	48	.47
Leading a healthy life	not effective	51	.43
Having sexual contact with fewer partners	lightly effective; not effective	52	.34
[Being careful] who you have sex with	slightly effective; not effective	54	.40
Taking the pill	not effective	86	.42
Not making love with people belonging to a risk group	lightly effective; not effective	29	.29
Holding off on love-making until you can trust the other person	not effective	31	.24
Washing yourself after you've made love with someone	not effective	71	.47

* alpha is .75.

APPENDIX B. Sexual permissiveness scale *

	% (completely) agree	item rest correlation
People should be allowed to go to bed with each other only when they have a steady relationship	40	.46
If you think about it, there's no excuse for masturbation	8	.54
Young people who know each other for just a short time, shouldn't go to bed together yet	43	.43
A man should always act like a man	39	.46
I find homosexuality (sexual contact between people of the same sex) a normal form of sexual expression	51	.59
It's alright when young boys also learn to knit in elementary school	51	.32
It would be better if the differences between men and women were to gradually disappear	70	.38
It's alright if a married woman retains her maiden name if she wants to	68	.47
In a steady relationship, you should allow each other to have sexual contact with a third person	5	.36
Even within a steady relationship, masturbation can be normal	60	.51

* alpha is .78.

APPENDIX C. Worries about general topics scale *

	mean	item rest correlation
That I'll get a venereal disease	1.2	.23
That I'll get a serious disease	1.9	.42
Loneliness	1.6	.32
Illness of a family member	2.4	.32
My health	2.2	.48
My outward appearance	1.8	.35
Becoming discriminated against	1.7	.31
My weight	2.1	.29
Smoking too much	1.9	.31
Drinking too much	1.5	.25
Difficulties with sex	1.4	.24
World-wide destruction of the environment	3.1	.33
Weapons of mass destruction throughout the world	2.5	.37
Having enough money every month	2.0	.26
Crime on the streets	2.7	.32

* alpha is .72.

Sexual Behaviour in Injecting Drug Users

Michael W. Ross, PhD, MPH
Alex Wodak, MB, BS, FRACP
Julian Gold, MB, BS

SUMMARY. This study examines the reported sexual behaviour of 1,245 injecting drug users (both in and out of treatment) who were recruited off the street in Sydney, Australia. The major differences in sexual behaviour were determined by sexual orientation (homosexual, bisexual or heterosexual). Condom use in the six months prior to interview was higher than that reported by IDUs in New York but similar to that reported in San Francisco and the U.K., with bisexual men reporting higher rates than heterosexual men, and homosexual men higher rates than bisexual men. Condom use for oral sex was low. Condom use with regular partners was about 5% lower than with casual partners. Regular partners of male IDUs were more likely not to be IDUs, with the converse true for women. Half the respondents were likely to be intoxicated when having sex. These data underline the importance of distinguishing between sexual orientation as well as gender in determining type and degree of risk associated with sexual behaviour in IDUs, and suggest that condom use should be assessed in terms of known risk behaviours

Michael W. Ross is affiliated with the National Centre in HIV Social Research, School of Community Medicine, University of New South Wales, Sydney. Alex Wodak is affiliated with the Alcohol and Drug Service, St Vincent's Hospital, Sydney. Julian Gold is affiliated with the Albion Street (AIDS) Centre, Sydney Hospital, Sydney.

Address correspondence to Dr. Michael Ross, National Centre in HIV Social Research, School of Community Medicine, University of New South Wales, 345 Crown Street, Surry Hills, NSW 2010, Australia.

This study was funded by a Commonwealth AIDS Research Grant and forms part of a national study of HIV infection risks in IDUs. The work of Michael Drury, Jill Thomas, Sal Renshaw, Peter Karlsson, Vivienne Griffin, Leslie Armstrong, Neil Carroll, Simon Nimmo, Helen Johns, Vanessa French and Paul Fleming on this study is gratefully acknowledged.

(vaginal and anal intercourse) rather than across all sexual contacts when sexual risk for HIV transmission is assessed.

While there has been considerable recent research on the nature and frequency of sexual risk behaviours for the purpose of determining the risk of Human Immunodeficiency Virus (HIV) infection among homosexual and bisexual males, there has been little research into sexual behaviour in other subgroups of the population apart from prisoners and sex workers. However, with concern over the increasing evidence of HIV transmission spreading beyond the major groups of people perceived as being at risk, more attention needs to be directed to the sexual behaviour within subcultures. Injecting drug users (IDUs) are of particular interest for several reasons including their potential double risk of HIV infection (through contaminated injection equipment and unprotected sex), the possibility of sexual activity or drug injecting occurring while intoxicated, and their status as a stigmatised and often covert minority group in western society. The recent evidence of uncontrolled spread of HIV infection among IDUs in developing countries (Des Jarlais, Choopanya, Wenston, Vanichseni, Sotheran & Plangsringarm, 1991) as well as developed countries adds an extra urgency to this field of research.

Control of sexual transmission in this population will also result in a reduction in vertical transmission which is a further important benefit. However, published research on the sexual behaviour of IDUs is scant, often only carried out as an adjunct to the study of drug injecting behaviour, and frequently methodologically flawed.

Most previous research into sexual behaviour in IDUs has focused on degree of sexual risk for HIV infection, although most are flawed by failure to distinguish between rates for males and females, across sexual orientation, and between personal and commercial sex. In New York City, Nemoto, Brown, Foster and Chu (1990) report that methadone clinic recruits were at high sexual risk (as only 11 to 14% used condoms) while Magura, Shapiro, Siddiqi and Lipton (1990) also found that only 11% of IDUs in the same city used condoms all the time in a similar population. In San Francisco, Lewis and Watters (1991) reported that in heterosexual male and female IDUs, two thirds never used condoms (with men using condoms less frequently than women). In the UK, Klee, Faugier, Hayes and Morris (1990) also found that three quarters of sexually active male and female IDUs never used condoms. A similar finding was reported by McKeganey, Barnard and Watson (1989) in Scotland, where 79% of IDUs interviewed were not using or not prepared to use condoms. A longitudinal study by Klee, Faugier, Hayes and Morris (1991) noted that while condom use in a sample of IDUs rose from 20% to 31% over nine months, their use was most likely to occur with the unattached who were probably the most sexually active. No reasons for the changes were provided. McKeganey et al. (1989) reported that the sexual partners for 84% of their sample were *not* drug injectors. As they point out, this makes probable the spread of HIV beyond IDUs highly probable particularly as IDUs were more concerned about the possibility of *contracting* HIV rather than *spreading* it to others.

Differences have also been reported in the likelihood of safer sexual behaviours between personal and commercial situations. In Amsterdam, van den Hoek, van Haastrecht and Couthino (1990) found that while 86% of female prostitutes used condoms with clients, only 20% used them with regular partners. Nor was there any difference between the frequency of condom use with regular and casual partners. On the other hand, Abdul-Quader, Tross, Friedman, Kouzi and Des Jarlais (1990) in New York City reported that 61% of their sample of male and female IDUs had deliberately decreased their sexual risk (with 44% now practicing safer sex including using condoms), and in Italy, Martin, Serpelloni, Galvan, Rizetto, Gomma, Morgante and Rezza (1990) found that an audiovisual presentation on HIV risks lead to a reported increase in condom use from 49 to 70% in male and female IDUs (and a decrease in needle and syringe sharing from 35% to 12%). These data suggest that IDUs are potentially responsive to interventions to reduce risk of HIV transmission. However, against this it must be noted that there are some data which suggest that IDUs may be at increased risk of HIV infection sexually compared to the general community. Ross, Gold, Wodak and Miller (1991) found that IDUs in Sydney had a very high lifetime prevalence of STDs. As genital ulcer disease is a co-factor in sexual transmission of HIV, an increased prevalence of STDs in IDUs will result in a higher risk of sexual transmission if condoms are not used. Although spread of HIV infection from IDUs to the rest of the community occurs by sexual transmission, it may be facilitated by STDs which appear to be prevalent in this population.

The purpose of this study was to assess the sexual practices of a large sample of Australian IDUs to both determine differences between regular and casual partners and to determine differences across sexual orientation and gender, both aspects given little attention in earlier research. Further, sexual behaviour in IDUs has previously not been described in sufficient detail to enable assessment of differences within this group.

METHOD

This study formed part of a national HIV-IDU research project. Sydney, the largest city in Australia with a population of almost four million in the greater urban area, is the capital of New South Wales and is considered the drug and prostitution capital of the south Pacific (Harcourt & Philpot, 1990). Respondents were obtained by three forms of advertising. First, by interviewers distributing cards with study details and the telephone and address of the interview site, and the indication that IDUs would be paid $A 20 for an anonymous interview; second, by putting advertisements with the same message in employment and social security offices, needle exchanges and pharmacies which sold needles and syringes; and third, by placing the same advertisement in a popular free central city magazine. Interviews took place in an unmarked building several blocks from the centre of the drug-using subculture in the Kings Cross-Darlinghurst area of Sydney, with direct access off the street into a waiting room. These interviews were conducted in an individual private cubicle by interviewers who had extensive personal or professional experience in the area of injecting drug use. A single receptionist recorded initials of first and surnames and date of birth and where respondents were suspected or recognized as having attended previously, these data were checked to ensure that there was no double interviewing. In addition, interviews were conducted by one interviewer in the western suburbs of Sydney to obtain a broader geographical distribution of injecting drug users: these interviews were conducted at a community health centre under the same conditions. All data were entered on the interview schedule by the interviewer. At the conclusion of the interview, respondents were invited to contribute a drop of blood obtained by Microlet[R] from the tip of the central digit on to a strip of blotting paper, which was then coded, dried and sealed in a plastic bag for laboratory analysis. Those respondents who had already reported a positive HIV test were not retested, following the approach of McCusker, Koblin, Lewis and Sullivan (1990). Payment took place at the completion of the interview preceding the blood collection to emphasise the voluntary nature of blood analysis. Because the dried (capillary) blood spot test is not as accurate as venous blood testing, results were not available to respondents. Those who expressed an interest in knowing their HIV status were directed to a clinic next door where appropriate pre- and post-test counselling was provided in conjunction with a standard venous blood test. Because of the anonymous and confidential nature of the procedure, there was no way of identifying those respondents who did test positive on the dried blood spot tests. Interviews were conducted between May and December 1989.

The study employed an interview schedule which had been piloted on over 100 injecting drug users and subsequently modified. Sections covered demographics, sexual history, drug use behaviour, use of new equipment/reuse of own equipment, sharing of injection equipment, cleaning of injection equipment, disposal of used injection equipment, social context of injecting drug use, knowledge and attitudes about HIV/AIDS, HIV/AIDS prevention behaviours, sources of HIV/AIDS information, HIV/AIDS antibody testing, and modules on treatment and prison use if appropriate. Response possibilities ranged from closed options to open-ended questions. All response possibilities were provided on show-cards where appropriate (a copy of the full 36 page interview schedule is available from the first author on request). The interview took on average 1 hour to complete.

RESULTS

Sample Characteristics. A total of 1,245 respondents who had injected drugs in the last two years were interviewed: these included 908 males, 331 females, and six male to female transsexuals (who have been excluded from this analysis). Characteristics of the males and females are described separately (means ± SDs are given where appropriate).

Mean age was 27.9 ± 6.7 for males (females 26.3 ± +7.6), and modal highest level of education was some high school (57.2% of the males, 53.5% of the female sample). Modal employment status was social security benefits or pension for 59.2% of males and 58.5% of females, with only 13.5% (16.7%) employed full- or part-time and 20.0% (13.7%) unemployed. The majority of males (50.8%) and females (57.6%) had been on benefits or pension for over one year, and a further 38.2% (32%) for over a month. The sample was predominantly Australian-born (79.2% of males, 84.6% of females) with the majority of the remainder (15.5% of males, 12.3% of females) being born in the UK, New Zealand, or North America. Mean number of children was 0.6 ± 1.3 for males, 0.9 ± 2.7 for females, with the mean number of children financially dependent on the respondent being 0.1 ± 0.5 (0.6 ± 2.1). The mean number of other people financially dependent on the respondent was 0.2 ± 2.6 for males and 0.1 ± 0.4 for females. Nearly half the males (45.2%) and less than a fifth of the females (19.6%) had been to prison, with a mean time of 3.6 ± 3.8 (4.9 ± 8.4) years since release. Just over half (55.4% of males, 54.1% of females) had moved to Sydney from elsewhere, on an average of 4.8 ± 7.7 (4.9 ± 8.4) years ago.

Drug Treatment. A majority of both males (63.8%) and females (55.9%) had been in some form of drug treatment, which had ended on average 2.3 ± 4.6 (2.3 ± 5.5) years ago. The most common previous treatments were Methadone maintenance (19.7% of males, 21% of females), detoxification (40.1% of males, 48.5% of females) and inpatient rehabilitation (13.0%) for males and counselling (10.2%) for females. For those currently in treatment (30.4% of males, 15.7% of females), the most common treatment was Methadone maintenance (39% of males and 49.1% of females) followed by therapeutic community (26.6% of males, 12% of females).

Drug Use. Most respondents were currently injecting with the majority having injected within hours (17.2% of males, 20.3% of females) or days (33.9% of males, 30.9% of females) of the interview: only 6.7% of males and 2.7% of females had not injected within the year. Mean age of first injection of a drug was 18.6 ± 4.4 years for males, 18.1 ± 3.8 for females, and mean age of injecting a drug once a month or more was 20.0 ± 4.6 (19.0 ± 4.4) years. Average frequency of injecting (or for those not currently injecting, when they were last injecting) per typical month was 49 ± 66 times for males, 53 ± 66 times for females. The drugs most commonly injected in the last typical using month (more than one could be nominated) were heroin (67.1% of males, 70.1% of females), amphetamines (34.6% of males, 32.2% of females) and cocaine (13.2% of the male and 15.1% of the female sample).

Sexual Behaviour. Comparisons of sexual behaviour of males and females and sexual orientation groups are presented in Tables 1 to 5. Eighty three males and 60 females reported being paid for sex (Table 5). Because of missing values, many of the *n*s will sum to less than the total *n*. Table 1 indicates that vaginal, oral and manual stimulation were the most common modes of sex for heterosexual and bisexual men, and the same holding for homosexual men with the exception of vaginal sex. However, anal sex was reported by less than half of the homosexual men in the past six months (and eight percent of the heterosexual men).

Table 2 illustrates the sexual behaviours engaged in by the women in the sample in the past six months. For heterosexual women, vaginal, oral and manual sex were again the most common practices, and for the lesbians, oral and manual sex were the most common. In pattern, the bisexual women were most similar to the heterosexual women.

Payment for sex was reported as having ever occurred in over one third of the homosexual and bisexual men but less than 5% of the heterosexual men, in about 10% of the homosexual and heterosexual women but in over one third of the bisexual women (Table 5).

Condom use for both males and females was higher in casual

TABLE 1

USUAL SEXUAL PRACTICES OF MALES, PERCENT

(PERCENT EVER ENGAGED)

Practice	Homosexual	Bisexual	Heterosexual
Vaginal intercourse	0 (16.0)	66.6 (78.6)	90.0 (90.3)
Vaginal intercourse (withdraw before orgasm)	0 (10.0)	18.0 (40.2)	12.3 (44.8)
Anal sex (give, without condom)	20.0 (44.0)	17.1 (36.8)	8.0 (20.8)
Anal sex (take, without condom)	22.0 (50.0)	13.7 (23.9)	0 (2.4)
Anal sex (give, with condom)	46.0 (64.0)	24.7 (38.5)	2.6 (6.6)
Anal sex (take, with condom)	42.0 (58.0)	17.1 (26.5)	0 (1.7)
Anal sex (take, withdraw before orgasm)	10.0 (18.0)	6.8 (12.8)	0 (2.8)
Anal sex (give, withdraw before orgasm)	14.0 (30.0)	7.7 (18.0)	0 (6.8)
Oral sex (give to man)	68.0 (80.0)	29.9 (47.9)	0 (2.5)
Oral sex (give to man, withdraw before orgasm)	58.0 (74.0)	19.7 (36.8)	0 (1.7)
Oral sex (give to woman)	0 (10.0)	57.3 (70.9)	57.9 (76.3)
Oral sex (taking it)	52.0 (66.0)	68.4 (53.9)	51.9 (67.7)
Manual stimulation (to man)	68.0 (80.0)	35.9 (53.9)	2.5 (6.2)
Manual stimulation (to woman)	2.0 (6.0)	53.9 (66.7)	57.8 (74.2)
Manual stimulation (take it)	60.0 (68.0)	51.3 (71.8)	42.6 (60.7)
Rimming	16.0 (38.0)	12.0 (29.9)	4.3 (10.1)
Fisting	2.0 (12.0)	3.4 (10.3)	0.1 (2.6)

TABLE 2

USUAL SEXUAL PRACTICES OF FEMALES, PERCENT

(PERCENT EVER ENGAGED)

Practice	Homosexual	Bisexual	Heterosexual
Vaginal intercourse	0 (60.0)	73.7 (87.4)	86.4 (98.6)
Vaginal intercourse (withdraw before orgasm)	0 (20.0)	13.7 (46.3)	17.7 (44.6)
Anal sex (take, without condom)	0 (10.0)	6.3 (27.4)	3.6 (23.6)
Anal sex (take, with condom)	0 (0)	4.2 (13.7)	2.3 (7.7)
Anal sex (take, withdraw before orgasm)	0 (0)	1.1 (9.5)	1.4 (10.9)
Oral sex (give to man)	0 (0)	54.7 (75.8)	55.0 (77.7)
Oral sex (give to man, withdraw before orgasm)	0 (0)	34.7 (65.3)	36.8 (59.6)
Oral sex (give to woman)	50.0 (60.0)	44.2 (71.6)	0 (7.2)
Oral sex (taking it)	50.0 (50.0)	73.7 (89.5)	54.6 (70.5)
Manual stimulation (to man)	0 (0)	37.9 (73.7)	47.3 (74.6)
Manual stimulation (to woman)	70.0 (70.0)	39.0 (72.6)	3.6 (10.5)
Manual stimulation (take it)	30.0 (30.0)	60.0 (81.1)	43.2 (65.0)
Rimming	20.0 (20.0)	3.2 (22.1)	5.0 (11.8)
Fisting	0 (0)	2.1 (5.3)	0.1 (5.0)

partners compared with regular partners (Tables 3 and 4) with higher figures for anal sex in homosexual men. In general, there was higher condom use for vaginal and anal sex than for oral sex. There were no differences across sexual orientation for women although a higher rate of condom use for casual partners was also reported.

Sexual Orientation. Sexual orientation was defined by sexual

TABLE 3

CONDOM USE WITH REGULAR PARTNERS IN MALES (%)

	Homosexual	Bisexual	Heterosexual	Sig*
All Partners				
Vaginal sex	0	40.8	30.9	Ho>He
Anal sex (giving it)	70.7	45.6	22.0	Ho>Bi>He
Anal sex (taking it)	75.6	58.4	0	He<Bi,Ho
Oral sex (giving it to a man)	22.4	31.5	0	Bi>He
Oral sex (taking it)	19.2	21.5	10.2	Bi>He
Regular Partner(s)				
Vaginal sex	0	35.0	22.4	Bi>He>Ho
Anal sex (giving it)	64.6	39.9	12.9	Ho>Bi>He
Anal sex (taking it)	71.3	41.9	0	Ho>Bi>He
Oral sex (taking it)	14.3	15.8	0	He<Ho,Bi
Oral sex (giving it)	13.7	18.2	11.6	ns

*p<.05

partners in the past five years with bisexuals reporting at least one sexual contact with males and females in this period. Group sizes for males were Homosexual 50, Bisexual 117, Heterosexual 719, and for females, Lesbian 10, Bisexual 95, and Heterosexual 220. There was a significant relationship between HIV status and sexual orientation in men ($X^2_2 = 77.6$, p < .001; Homosexual 35.4%, Bisexual 12.1%, Heterosexual 3.2%) and in women ($X^2_2 = 17.3$, p < .001; Lesbian 42.9%, Bisexual 3.8%, Heterosexual 5.7%). Of all those HIV positive, 14 were detected by dried blood spot analysis and the remainder (50) by self-report (49 males, 15 females). The number of HIV tests performed per respondent differed significantly between sexual orientation groups for both men and women (respectively, $X^2_2 = 16.8$, p < .001, Heterosexual 76.2%, Bisexual 88.8%, Homosexual 94%; $X^2_2 = 6.4$, p < .05, Heterosexual 73.4%, Bisexual 86.3%, Lesbian 80.0%). Having an HIV test was reported

TABLE 4

CONDOM USE WITH REGULAR PARTNERS IN FEMALES (%)

	Heterosexual	Bisexual	Sig*
All Partners			
Vaginal sex	37.1	45.0	ns
Anal sex (taking it)	41.0	19.6	ns
Oral sex (giving it to a man)	15.4	26.2	ns
Regular Partners			
Vaginal sex	22.4	26.1	ns
Anal sex (taking it)	20.6	14.4	
Oral sex (giving it to a man)	8.2	9.5	

*p<.05

by male respondents to have changed their sexual behaviour (X^2_2 = 9.8, p < .01; Homosexual 59.6%, Bisexual 60.4%, Heterosexual 45.9%) but this was not true for females (X^2_2 = 2.2, ns; Lesbian 25%, Bisexual 51.9%, Heterosexual 47.6%).

Sexual Partners. Mean number of sexual partners reported by male respondents over the past year reported was for male partners, Homosexual 23.1, Bisexual 10.8 (F_2 = 49.0, p < .001), and for female partners, Heterosexual 6.1, Bisexual 6.2, Homosexual 0 (F_2 = 3.7, p < .05). For female respondents, mean number of sexual partners was for male partners, Heterosexual 8.1, Bisexual 28.1, Lesbian 0 (F_2 = 1.9, ns), and for female partners, Heterosexual 0, Bisexual 4.2, Lesbian 4.2 (F_2 = 12.2, p < .001). The proportion who had a regular partner who was bisexual was significantly different across sexual orientation for both sexes (males, Heterosexual 9.1%, Bisexual 46.4%, Homosexual 18.8%, X^2_2 = 71.1, p < .001; females, Heterosexual 3.9%, Bisexual 30.1%, Lesbians, 0%, X^2_2 = 36.8, p < .001).

Drug Use and Sexual Behaviour. Proportion of male respondents who had a regular partner(s) who injected drugs was, Heterosexual 55.9%, Bisexual 58.3%, Homosexual 18.8% (X^2_2 = 2.1, ns), and for

TABLE 5

PAYMENT FOR SEX IN INJECTING DRUG USERS

(% in brackets)

	Homosexual	Bisexual	Heterosexual
Males Paid for Sex:	38.8% (16)	33.9% (39)	4.0% (28)[*]
Of those paid, frequency:			
Less than once/year	3	12	10
1-3 times/month	7	14	15
1-6 times/week	3	4	3
>7 times/week	3	9	0
Regular form of income:	6	13	7
Females Paid for Sex:	10.0% (1)	35.2% (32)	12.6% (27)[*]
Of those paid, frequency:			
Less than once/year	1	3	7
1-3 times/month	0	9	7
1-6 times/week	0	6	3
>7 times/week	0	14	6
Regular form of income:	0	20	17

female respondents, Heterosexual 78.3%, Bisexual 69.3%, Lesbian 62.5% ($X^2_2 = 3.0$, ns). The proportion of occasions that respondents reported being "high, stoned or drunk" when having sex was for males, Heterosexual 57.8, Bisexual, 59.1, Homosexual, 58.9 ($F_2 = 0.2$, ns) and for females, Lesbian 54.7, Bisexual 66.0, and Heterosexual, 53.1 ($F_2 = 7.0$, p < .001).

DISCUSSION

The representativeness of samples of IDUs is problematic as the size and characteristics of the drug-using population in a community has never been defined confidently. However, this is a large sample, recruited systematically, and the demographic characteristics are comparable with other studies of IDUs in Australia. Self-report of sexual behaviours (McLaws, Oldenburg, Ross & Cooper, 1990) and drug use behaviours (Darke, Hall, Weather, Ward & Wodak, 1991) in IDUs has been demonstrated to be of acceptable reliability and validity. Although reliability and validity may be an additional source of error, this is unlikely to result in systematic bias. Because this is a cross-sectional study, temporal associations between the dependent and the independent variables cannot be estimated, and the effect of excluding cases with missing data (those who reported no sexual activity in the past five years to allow them to be classified according to sexual orientation, or sexual activity on the past six months on the sexual history) is unknown. Further, this study, in common with most other published studies on sexual behaviour in IDUs, lacks a control group of comparable non-IDUs, so that comparisons with frequency and safety of sexual activity in peers cannot be made. We have specifically compared across sexual orientation on risk behaviours in this sample, and have described the findings elsewhere (Ross, Wodak, Gold & Miller, in press).

With these caveats, the data indicate that sexual behaviour in Australian IDUs does show a range of differences across sexual orientation. First, the data indicate that for heterosexual males and females, vaginal intercourse is the most common sexual activity reported and that oro-genital and manual stimulation are also very common. There was a strong degree of concordance between proportions reported for oral and vaginal sex between males and females, although women reported less anal sex than men. For homosexual males, manual stimulation was the most common sexual activity reported, followed by oro-genital stimulation and anal intercourse. While not strictly comparable, these data for homosexually active men are similar to data reported by Ross (1986) in a study carried out in 1978 before the recognition of AIDS and suggest that the frequency of mutual masturbation appears to have increased while the frequency of oro-genital sex has decreased and the frequency of anal intercourse is unchanged.

However, condom use in the six months prior to interview is higher than that reported by IDUs in New York by Nemoto et al. (1990) and Magura et al. (1990) for vaginal sex in heterosexual men, but similar to that described in the U.K. and in San Francisco.

However, the figures for protected intercourse in this study are higher than those in the literature for the bisexual men in this study and higher still for the homosexual men. This indicates that it is important not to give an *overall* figure for condom use, but to differentiate both sexual orientation and type of sex. As an example, oro-genital sex is one of the most common sexual activities across the sample, but there is low condom use reported for this activity (possibly because of its apparently lower risk).

The differentiation between regular partners and casual partners in this study appears to result in a decrease of around 5% of frequency of condom use for sex (although this will also depend on the ratio between casual and regular partners). It should be noted that in Table 1, sexual behaviour in heterosexual males includes male-to-male manual sex, which is technically "homosexual." This suggests that heterosexual male IDUs in this sample may see sex as involving penetrative sex only, and makes it important to define what is meant by "sex" at the commencement of any study.

Homosexual and bisexual IDUs reported more HIV tests. This probably reflects an increased perception of greater risk through their sexual orientation. HIV status also reflected differences in sexual orientation, with a tenfold increase in prevalence of HIV infection among homosexual male IDUs as compared with heterosexual male IDUs. However, this latter finding is probably related to the fact that HIV infection in Australia is associated primarily with homosexually active men. Thus much of the HIV infection in the men in this sample is likely to have resulted from sexual risk rather than drug-related risk. However, given the few reported cases of lesbian sexual HIV transmission, for lesbians most of the transmission is likely to have been from injecting drug use. These data also emphasise the importance of considering sexual risk behaviours as means of HIV transmission in IDUs and of not making the assumption that HIV transmission in IDUs is primarily through drug use.

As in other studies, the regular sexual partners of male IDUs were more likely to not be IDUs themselves, although partners of female IDUs were more likely to be IDUs. However, this relationship appears to hold mainly for heterosexual and bisexual relationships in men and women as homosexual male IDUs were less likely to have IDU partners. Again, these data highlight the importance of analysing sexual behaviour in IDUs by sexual orientation and sexual act, given the significantly different patterns of sexual risk behaviour across these variables. Bisexual males and females were also more likely to have bisexual partners. While there were no differences in the proportion of the time respondents were intoxicated when having sex for men, the bisexual women were more likely to be intoxicated when having sex, possibly because more of them worked in the sex industry. Nevertheless, the fact that more than half of all respondents were intoxicated when having sex is an important finding as this will probably increase the likelihood of unsafe sexual practices. This needs to be taken into account when attempting to alter risk behaviours. In summary, these data demonstrate that the levels of unprotected sexual contact in IDUs are highest in heterosexual IDUs, and that they are much lower for homosexual and bisexual men. However, no assessment of actual level of risk can be made on actual risk levels, as we have no data on the number of sexual acts which occurred, although we do have data on number of partners and sexual act. When the pattern of sexual activity is examined, it is apparent that some of the most common sexual activities are those with low or no risk of HIV transmission such as oral sex or manual sex. Discussion of protected sex must thus be specific with regard to the activity.

These data also demonstrate that a sizeable proportion of IDUs have used condoms. Condom use in this study was commoner than reported in some overseas studies. Further, the gap between condom use with regular and other partners is less than reported in other studies. It would be appropriate to build on this base of use in future education campaigns.

REFERENCES

Abdul-Quader AS, Tross S, Friedman SR, Kouzi AC, Des Jarlais DC. (1990) Street-recruited intravenous drug users and sexual risk reduction in New York City. *AIDS* 4:1075-1079.

Darke S, Hall W, Heather N, Ward J, Wodak A. (1991) The reliability and validity of a scale to measure HIV risk-taking behaviour amongst intravenous drug users. *AIDS* 5:181-185.

Des Jarlais DC, Choopanya K, Wenston J, Vanichseni S, Sotheran JL, Plangsrin-garm K. (1991) Risk reduction and stabilization of HIV seroprevalence among drug injectors in New York City and Bangkok, Thailand. Abstract. MC1, Seventh International Conference on AIDS, Florence, Italy.

Harcourt C, Philpot R. (1990) Female prostitutes, AIDS, drugs and alcohol in NSW. In: Plant, M (ed) *AIDS, Drugs and Prostitution*. Routledge: London, 132-158.

Klee H, Faugier J, Hayes C, Boulton T, Morris J. (1990) Factors associated with risk behaviour among injecting drug users. *AIDS Care* 2:133-145.

Klee H, Faugier J, Hayes C, Morris J. (1991) Risk reduction among injecting drug users: changes in the sharing of injecting equipment and in condom use. *AIDS Care, 3*:63-73.

Lewis DK, Watters JK. (1991) Sexual risk behaviour among heterosexual intravenous drug users: ethnic and gender variations. *AIDS 5*:77-83.

McCusker J, Koblin B, Lewis BF, Sullivan J. (1990) Demographic characteristics, risk behaviors, and HIV seroprevalence among intravenous drug users by site of contact: results from a community-wide HIV surveillance project. *American Journal of Public Health* 80:1062-1067.

McKeganey N, Barnard M, Watson H. (1989) HIV-related risk behaviour among a non-clinic sample of injecting drug users. *British Journal of Addiction 84*:1481-1490.

McLaws ML, Oldenburg B, Ross MW, Cooper DA. (1990) Sexual behaviour in AIDS-related research: reliability and validity of recall and diary measures. *Journal of Sex Research* 27:265-281.

Magura S, Shapiro JL, Siddiqi Q, Lipton DS. (1990) Variables influencing condom use among intravenous drug users. *American Journal of Public Health 80*:82-84.

Martin GS, Serpelloni G, Galvan U, Rizzetto A, Gomma M, Morgante S, Rezza G. (1990) Behavioural change in injecting drug users: evaluation of an HIV/AIDS education programme. *AIDS Care* 2:275-279.

Nemoto T, Brown LS, Foster K, Chu A. (1990) Behavioral risk factors of Human Immunodeficiency Virus infection among intravenous drug users and implications for preventive interventions. *AIDS Education and Prevention* 2:116-126.

Ross MW. (1986) *Psychovenereology*. New York: Praeger.

Ross MW, Gold J, Wodak A, Miller ME. (1991) Sexually transmissible diseases in injecting drug users. *Genitourinary Medicine* 67:32-36.

Ross MW, Wodak A, Gold J, Miller ME. (1992) Differences across sexual orientation on HIV risk behaviours in injecting drug users. *AIDS Care 4*:in press.

van den Hoek JAR, van Haastricht HJA, Couthino RA. (1989) Heterosexual behaviour of intravenous drug users in Amsterdam: implications for the AIDS epidemic. *AIDS 4*:449-453.

Awareness of HIV Seropositivity and Psychosocial Factors Influence on the Sexual Contact Pattern: A Population Study of HIV-Infected Homosexual Men, in the City of Malmö, Sweden

Leif Persson, BA
Bertil S. Hanson, MD
Per-Olof Östergren, MD
Torkil Moestrup, MD
Sven-Olof Isacsson, MD

SUMMARY. The objective of this article was to describe a representative city population of HIV antibody positive homosexual and bisexual men regarding their psychosocial situation, and to examine if awareness of their seropositivity and different psychosocial factors influenced the sexual contact pattern. The population consists of all detected HIV seropositive homosexual and bisexual men who did not have an AIDS-diagnosis, and who were in contact with the only clinic in Malmö caring for seropositive individuals. Forty-seven gay men (72%) participated in the study during a one-year period from April 1988 when the population was defined. All men were inter-

Leif Persson, Bertil S. Hanson, and Per-Olof Östergren are affiliated with the Department of Community Health Sciences; Torkil Moestrup is affiliated with the Department of Infectious Diseases; and Sven-Olof Isacsson is affiliated with the Department of Community Health Sciences. All five authors are at Lund University, Malmö.

This study has been granted by the Swedish Medical Research Council.

Address correspondence to Leif Persson, Department of Health Sciences, Lund University, Malmö General Hospital, S-214 01 Malmö, Sweden.

viewed with a structured questionnaire and examined by a physician. The questionnaire contained items on psychosocial factors like social network, social support, stressful life events, health status, sexual orientation, and sexual contact patterns.

After awareness of seropositivity there was a decrease in both the number of ways of making sexual contacts and in the number of new sexual contacts. Men who had contact with HIV, gay or other organisations or a counsellor more often had possibilities of making sexual contacts and also more often made new sexual contacts after awareness of seropositivity. To have social, emotional and sexual contacts is important for an individual's self-esteem and psychological well-being. Psychosocial resources like contacts with organisations and counsellors give a person possibilities to handle stressful situations in life and to resist tendencies of social isolation. This is essential for health, and might even be of importance for the progression of the HIV-infection.

Human immunodeficiency virus (HIV) has become a great challenge for the international community. Efforts have been made to understand the natural history of the HIV infection and to develop drugs to treat the infection and its severe complications. Knowledge of psychosocial factors is crucial in order to obtain and to maintain behavioral changes among people at risk (Coates, McKusick, Kuno & Stites, 1989), but also to give good care and support to those already infected (Chuang, Devins, Hunsley & Gill, 1989; Ostrow, Monjan, Joseph, Raden, Fox et al., 1989).

Sexual behavior among gay men has been the objective of many studies with the goal of increasing the efficiency of prevention. Attention has mostly been directed towards sexual techniques and the use of condoms (Ekstrand & Coates, 1990; Roffman, Gilmore, Gilchrist, Mathias & Krueger, 1990). In contrast to these studies, this study in the field of social epidemiology, focuses on *sexual contact patterns*. This concept refers here to whether an individual makes any new sexual contacts and, if so, at what kinds of places, and how often new sexual contacts are made. The focus is on sexual contact patterns rather than on sexual behaviors since sexual contacts here are seen as a part of social network and social support. Various studies focus on the influence of psychosocial factors such as social network and social support on changes in risky sexual behavior. These latter studies present, however, contradictory results. In a New York study gay men practicing risky sex had better emotional support (Siegel, Mesagno, Chen & Christ, 1989). In a San Francisco study participants who had a large number of people on whom they could rely for social support were less likely to practice risky sex (Ekstrand & Coates, 1990). A study from Michigan showed that gay social network affiliation was not related to behavioral change in homosexual men (Emmons, Joseph, Kessler, Wortman, Montgomery et al., 1986).

The diagnosis of HIV may lead to a social and emotional withdrawal from social life (Siegel & Krauss, 1991). This could imply a loss of important psychosocial resources sorely needed when coping with the existential crisis and stressful situation of being HIV infected. To be able to maintain, or even to improve one's social support after awareness of seropositivity, can be essential for the well-being of an individual and perhaps also for the progression of the infection (Prieur, 1990). Various non-HIV related studies do show the importance of having good social network and social support in order to prevent social isolation and thus the impact of stress (Hanson, 1988).

The largest group in the United States, northern Europe and other industrialized parts of the world that has been infected with HIV is men who have sex with men (WHO, 1989). Most studies of homosexual men are, however, based on populations that have been enrolled at STD clinics, at gay meeting places or through advertisements in papers and magazines (McKusick, Coates, Morin, Pollack & Hoff, 1990). These populations may not be representative of the general population of HIV seropositive gay men and that constitutes a major problem when generalizing the results from these studies. This fact could to some part explain earlier inconsistencies.

The objective of this study is, therefore, to describe a representative city population of HIV antibody positive self-defined homosexual and bisexual men, regarding their psychosocial situation, and to examine if and how awareness of their seropositivity and different psychosocial factors influence their sexual contact patterns.

STUDY POPULATION

This homosexual and bisexual male population study in Malmö, Sweden, is a part of a prospective study of the influence of different psychosocial factors on the HIV progression. Malmö is a city in southern Sweden with about 230,000 inhabitants. The Department of Infectious Diseases at Malmö General Hospital is the only hospital clinic in the city that takes care of HIV infected patients. Almost all patients who are detected at other clinics are transferred to the Department of Infectious Diseases for care and treatment. Therefore, almost all known HIV seropositive homosexual and bisexual men in Malmö are in contact with this clinic.

The population of this cross-sectional study was defined in 1988/89. The total number of known HIV seropositive persons in Malmö in December 1988 was 136; of those, 91 were homosexual and bisexual men (Table 1). Of all people diagnosed with AIDS during recent years in Malmö, two thirds were already known as seropositive patients at the Department of Infectious Diseases (Hansson H-B, 1991). This fact indicates that the unknown proportion of HIV seropositive homosexual and bisexual men in Malmö is smaller than in many other countries and that the 91 known seropositive homosexual and bisexual men form a rather large part of all HIV seropositive homosexual and bisexual men in Malmö.

The population of this study consists of all detected HIV seropositive homosexual and bisexual men. To be included in the study the men should not be diagnosed with AIDS by CDC classification (CDC, 1986), and they had to be in contact with the Department of Infectious Diseases in Malmö during the one-year period from April

Table 1

Number and percentage of detected HIV infected persons in Malmö in December 1988.

	HIV Infected	thereof with AIDS
Homo- and bisexual men	91 (67%)	14
Intravenous drug abusers	14 (10%)	0
Persons infected by blood-products	16 (12%)	3
Persons infected heterosexually	14 (10%)	3
Persons with unknown transmission	1 (1%)	0
TOTAL	136 (100%)	20

1988 to April 1989. During that year, 90 HIV infected homo- and bisexual men had contact with the Department. One of the 91 seropositive gay men in Malmö was in contact with a physician outside the Department of Infectious Diseases. Fourteen of these 90 men were diagnosed with AIDS (CDC, 1986). Eleven men had been tested anonymously and were not in contact with the department during the year when the population was defined. They could therefore not be reached and asked to join the study. These 25 men were not included in the study population which therefore consists of 65 men.

METHODS

All men were interviewed consecutively with a structured questionnaire by one of two counsellors or one physician. In order to standardize the interviews the three interviewers discussed the questionnaire in advance and also made pilot interviews. The questionnaire contained items on psychosocial factors like aspects of social network and social support and stressful life-events, depression, stress experience, but also on sexual orientation, and sexual contact patterns. The basic parts (social network and social support) of this instrument have been elaborated in Malmö at the Department of Community Health Sciences, and have there been used in various population studies (Hanson & Östergren, 1987). The items measuring different aspects of social network and social support have proved to have a sufficient internal consistency and validity and a high reliability when tested (Hanson, 1988; Hanson, Isacsson, Janzon & Lindell, 1990).

Symptoms of the HIV-infection according to the CDC classification (CDC, 1986) were recorded in a standardized way at a clinical examination, one or several times during the study period. At these clinical examinations the amount of CD-4 lymphocytes /µl was also assessed in a standardized way (Reinherz & Schlossman, 1980).

Patient records were used to obtain information about months of awareness of the seropositivity, in-patient and out-patient care at the Department of Infectious Diseases and also to characterize the non-participants (Table 2).

Table 2

Characteristics of participants and non-participants (number and percentage). All continuous variables have been dichotomized at the median. (The differences are not statistically significant).

	Participants n=47	Non-participants n=18
Age		
≤39 years	29 (62 %)	8 (44 %)
>39 years	18 (38%)	10 (56%)
Social group		
White collar workers	24 (51 %)	8 (44 %)
Blue collar workers	23 (49%)	10 (56%)
Ethnic group		
Swedish	35 (74 %)	13 (72 %)
Immigrants	12 (26%)	5 (28%)
Awareness of seropositivity for HIV		
≤ 43 months	22 (47 %)	11 (61 %)
> 43 months	25 (53%)	7 (39%)
Out-patient care		
≤ 6 visits per year	22 (47 %)	11 (61 %)
> 6 visits per year	25 (53%)	7 (39%)
In-patient care		
yes	16 (34%)	7 (39%)
no	31 (66 %)	11 (61 %)
Symptoms of the HIV infection		
yes	19 (40%)	6 (33%)
no	28 (60 %)	12 (67 %)
CD-4 lymphocytes		
≤ 416/µl	24 (51%)	12 (67%)
> 416/µl	23 (49 %)	6 (33 %)

DEFINITIONS

Background Factors

The classification of social class is based on the individual's profession, working tasks and position. *Blue collar workers* are defined as skilled and unskilled workers (social class III), and *white collar workers* include middle-range civil servants and employees (social class II) and persons in leading positions, professionals with university degrees and owners of business enterprises with employees (social class I) (Carlsson, 1958). *Immigrants* are defined as those men who were born abroad.

Sexual Contact Patterns

The study participants were asked *at what places* they used to make sexual contacts, and *how often* they had sex when making *new sexual contacts* per month in the most typical way, before and after awareness of their seropositivity. In the analysis eight different ways of making sexual contacts were divided into two categories, four *social ways* and four *anonymous ways*. These various ways represent two means of satisfying partly different needs. The social ways may offer a wider sphere of contact, i.e., not only sexually but also socially and emotionally. Thus the social ways can be seen as potentially more rewarding in providing more advantageous psychosocial resources. The *social ways* of making sexual contact includes contacts at a gay bar/discotheque, a bar/discotheque for the general population, in social life (private parties) and advertisements in papers and magazines. The *anonymous ways* of making sex-contacts include contacts at saunas/porno-cinemas, at public toilets, when "cruising" (outdoors in parks, etc.) and through the "contact line" (a public telephone line for anonymous four-part calls often used for making sex contacts).

In the analysis of sexual contact patterns in different subgroups, the number of *new sexual contacts* in the men's habitual way after awareness of seropositivity was dichotomized between those men with and those men without any new sexual contacts. In the same way *the number of ways* of making sexual contacts, both social and anonymous, after awareness of seropositivity was dichotomized between those men who had some ways of making sexual contacts and those who had not.

Health Status

Firstly, health was assessed according to the presence of any *symptoms* of the HIV infection during the one-year period. The study population was in the analysis dichotomized into men *with symptoms* (CDC-classification III-IV) and men *without symptoms* (CDC-classification II) (CDC, 1986).

Secondly, the amount of CD-4 lymphocytes was measured at every physical examination and the mean value was calculated. In the analysis the distribution of CD-4 lymphocytes was dichotomized at the median ($416/\mu l$).

Additionally, experience of depression and of stress was assessed. The questionnaire contained the items "Have you been depressed lately?" and "Have you been under stress lately?"

Psychosocial Factors

An individual's *social network* (social ties in a *structural* sense) and *social support* (a *function* of the individual's interaction with his social network) are considered to be important psychosocial resources in the process of coping with demands and different stressful situations in daily life (Cassel, 1976; Hanson & Östergren, 1987). Important aspects to be studied of HIV-infected gay men are for example the number of close friends, to have a partner, to be a member of or to have contact with organisations, and to have contact with a counsellor.

Being together is in this study defined as cohabiting with a friend or a partner or having a partner without cohabiting. *Being alone* is defined as not cohabiting and not having a partner. Being a member of *an organisation* is defined as being a member of any type of organisation but not a gay organisation. *A gay organisation* is defined as an organisation for gay rights. A *voluntary HIV organisation* is defined as an HIV support and information organisation, an organisation of HIV infected persons, or a gay HIV support organisation.

The sexual orientation was assessed by a visual analogue scale through a marking somewhere on a line with two endpoints representing homosexuality and heterosexuality. A mark at the endpoint of homosexuality is defined as being *exclusively homosexual*. All marks somewhere on the line between the endpoints are defined as *not exclusively homosexual*.

Items on *stressful life-events* were included in the questionnaire and covered serious illness and deaths among close friends or relatives and experience of unemployment caused by HIV or something else.

Statistical Methods

Chi-square analysis was used to analyze differences between participants and non-participants and also in the count of CD-4 cells among men with and without symptoms, to analyze differences in sexual orientation between men who had and had not told their parents about the homosexuality and seropositivity and between the non-participant and participant groups. Chi-square analysis was also used to analyze differences in the sexual contact pattern before and after awareness of seropositivity. Odds ratios and 95% confidence intervals were used to analyse differences between groups of men with and without new sexual contacts (Table 3) and between groups of men with and without social or anonymous ways of making sexual contact (Table 4). Correlations between independent variables were estimated by the Pearson correlations coefficient (Table 5).

RESULTS

Analysis of the Non-Participants

Of the 65 men in the study population, 10 did not respond to the invitation to take part in the study and 8 men stated that they did not want to participate. Thus, 47/65 (72%) men participated. In order to analyze whether the participants were representative of the study population the following eight variables were analyzed for both participants and non participants: age, social class, nationality, number of months of awareness of their seropositivity, number of visits per year to the HIV clinic at the Department of Infectious Diseases, in-patient care at the Department for Infectious Diseases since awareness of seropositivity and health status. Rather small differences were found between participants and non-participants and the differences were not statistically significant (Table 2).

Table 3

The odds ratios (95 % confidence interval) of making new sexual contacts in
the habitual way in different groups in comparison with men who did not make
any new sexual contacts after awareness of HIV infection

	New sexual contacts (n=19)	No new sexual contacts (n=26)	Odds ratio (C I)
Age older/younger	13/6	10/16	3.5 (1.0-12)
Social Group white/blue collar	11/8	11/15	1.9 (0.6-6.2)
Ethnic Group Swedish/immigrant	13/6	20/6	0.7 (0.2-2.5)
Being Together yes/no	13/6	13/13	2.2 (0.6-7.4)
Close Friends many/few	12/7	14/12	1.5 (0.4-4.9)
Member of any Organization yes/no	7/12	4/22	3.2 (0.8-13)
Member of Gay Organization yes/no	14/5	10/16	4.5 (1.3-16)
Contact with Voluntary HIV Organization yes/no	10/9	9/17	2.1 (0.6-7.0)
Using Counselling yes/no	12/7	9/17	3.2 (0.96-11)
Experiencing Stress yes/no	14/5	17/9	1.5 (0.4-5.4)
Feeling Depressed yes/no	9/10	15/11	0.7 (0.2-2.2)

Table 4

The odds ratios (95 % confidence interval) of having <u>social</u> or <u>anonymous ways</u> of making sexual contacts, in different groups, in comparison with men who did not have any ways of making sexual contacts, after awareness of HIV infection

	Social Ways			Anonymous Ways		
	yes n=27	no n=20	Odds ratio (C I)	yes n=14	no n=33	Odds ratio (C I)
Age older/younger	12/15	12/8	0.5 (0.2-1.7)	8/6	16/17	1.4 (0.4-5.0)
Social Group white/blue collar	16/11	7/13	2.7 (0.8-8.8)	8/6	15/18	1.6 (0.5-5.6)
Ethnic Group Swedish/immigrant	20/7	15/5	1.0 (0.3-3.6)	11/3	24/9	1.4 (0.3-6.1)
Being Together yes/no	18/9	10/10	2.0 (0.6-6.5)	9/5	19/14	1.3 (0.4-4.8)
Close Friends many/few	14/13	14/6	0.5 (0.1-1.6)	8/6	20/13	0.9 (0.2-3.1)
Member of any Organization yes/no	9/18	3/17	2.8 (0.7-12)	7/7	5/28	5.6 (1.5-22)
Member of Gay Organization yes/no	18/9	7/13	3.7 (1.1-12)	13/1	12/21	23 (4.1-128)
Contact with Voluntary HIV Organization yes/no	14/13	6/14	2.5 (0.8-8.4)	10/4	10/23	5.8 (1.5-21)
Using Counselling yes/no	15/12	6/14	2.9 (0.9-9.7)	9/5	12/21	3.2 (0.9-11.3)
Experiencing Stress yes/no	21/6	11/9	2.9 (0.8-10)	12/2	20/13	3.9 (0.8-19)
Feeling Depressed yes/no	15/12	10/10	1.3 (0.4-4.0)	8/6	17/16	1.3 (0.4-4.4)

Table 5
Correlation analysis between the independent variables

	1	2	3	4	5	6	7	8	9	10	11
1) Age (< 37 years=1 ≥ 37 years=2)											
2) Social Class (white collar=1 blue collar=2)	.06 p=.34										
3) Ethnic Group (Swedish=1 immigrant=2)	-.01 p=.47	.09 p=.29									
4) Being Together (yes=1 no=2)	.11 p=.23	.29 p=.03	-.18 p=.11								
5) Close Friends (1=many 2=few)	.04 p=.40	.24 p=.05	-.09 p=.27	.36 p=.006							
6) Member of any Organization (yes=1 no=2)	.01 p=.47	.40 p=.002	.23 p=.06	.28 p=.03	.09 p=.27						
7) Member of Gay Organization (yes=1 no=2)	-.11 p=.24	.15 p=.16	.23 p=.06	-.16 p=.14	-.12 p=.22	.35 p=.007					
8) Contact with Voluntary HIV Organization (yes=1 no=2)	.02 p=.45	.02 p=.45	.01 p=.47	.008 p=.48	-.13 p=.18	.38 p=.004	.38 p=.005				
9) Using Counseling (yes=1 no= 2)	.06 p=.34	.15 p=.16	-.16 p=.14	.04 p=.39	.09 p=.27	.06 p=.34	.33 p=.01	.35 p=.008			
10) Experiencing Stress (yes=1 no=2)	.21 p=.08	-.06 p=.34	-.19 p=.10	-.01 p=.25	-.16 p=.14	-.02 p=.45	-.002 p=.50	.31 p=.02	.25 p=.05		
11) Feeling Depressed (yes=1 no=2)	-.02 p=.45	-.11 p=.24	.04 p=.40	.10 p=.26	-.02 p=.46	.16 p=.14	-.11 p=.23	.46 p=.001	.07 p=.32	.46 p=.001	

CHARACTERISTICS OF THE PARTICIPANTS

Demographics

The mean age of the 47 participants was 37 years (SD ± 7.61 years). The youngest was 23 and the oldest 53 years old (Figure 1). While twenty-three men (49%) were blue collar workers, the others were white collar workers. Twenty-eight men (60%) had a partner or cohabited either with the partner or a friend and the rest were alone. Twelve (26%) men were immigrants. Of these, five came from Scandinavia, three from other European countries and four from North or South America. Nineteen men (40%) described themselves as exclusively homosexual, while 28/47 (60%) did not (Figure 2).

HIV-Status

The mean number of months of the men's awareness of their seropositivity was 37 (SD ± 15), with a range of 5-55 months. Date of infection was known with rather good authenticity for 27/47 (57%) of the men. The mean time since seroconversion for these 27 men was 46 months (SD ± 6 months), with a range of 12-109 months. Eighteen men (38%) had HIV-related symptoms of which 12 also had a low count of CD-4 lymphocytes (below the median 416/µl), and only 6 had a high count ($p = 0.09$).

Stress, Depression and Stressful Life-Events

Of the 47 participants, 32 (68%) men reported experience of stress and 25 (47%) depression. Of the 32 men who reported experience of stress, 22 also reported experience of depression ($p = 0.002$). Twenty-two of the men who reported stressful life-events during the last year had had some of their nearest friends or relatives seriously ill during the last year. Twelve of these had been diagnosed with AIDS. Sixteen men (34%) had experienced deaths among their nearest relatives or friends, of whom nine had died of AIDS. Due to their HIV-infection six individuals had been forced

Figure 1.

The age distribution of the 47 homosexual and bisexual men

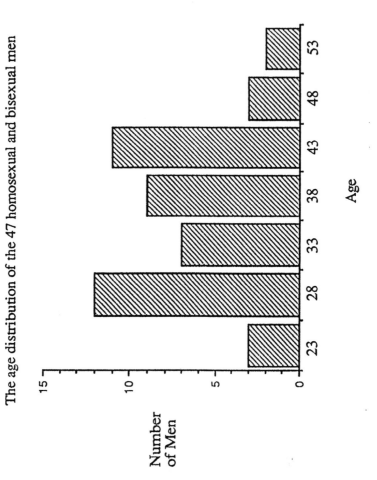

Figure 2.

Distribution of the sexual orientation among the 47 participating homo- and bisexual men

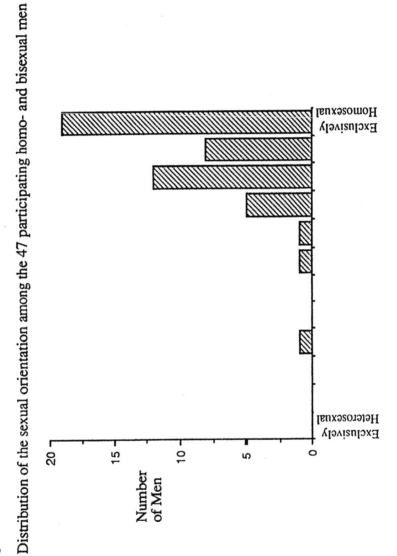

to change jobs and five of them also reported a severe conflict at their work due to the seropositivity. There was no statistical significant difference in reported experience of stress between those men who had experienced such stressful life-events and those who had not.

Social Network

The forty-seven men had a median of two heterosexual (Range 0-17) and three homosexual close friends (Range 0-13). More than twice as many homosexual as heterosexual friends knew about their seropositivity. Fourteen men reported that none of their heterosexual friends were informed about their HIV-status. Five of the participants had no homosexual friends who knew. Those men who described themselves as exclusively homosexual had, to a higher degree than the non-exclusively homosexual men, told their fathers about their homosexuality (80% compared to 48%, p = 0.05) and about their seropositivity (40% compared to 10%, p = 0.03). There was no statistical significant difference between the groups in telling their mothers.

In the studied group, twelve men (26%) were members of one or more organizations (other than gay or voluntary HIV organization), 26 men (55%) were members of a gay organization and 20 men (43%) had contact with a voluntary HIV organization. Twenty-one of the 47 men (45%) had contact with a counsellor.

Sexual Contact Patterns

The mean number of *ways of making sexual contacts* decreased after the men became aware of their seropositivity (Figure 3 and 4). Before awareness the mean number of *social ways* of making sexual contact was 2.2 (SD ± 1.1) and afterwards only 0.9 (SD ± 0.9), (p < 0.001). The mean number of *anonymous ways* was before awareness 1.5 (SD ± 1.2) and afterwards 0.5 (SD ± 0.9), (p < 0.001). One third (15 men) had only social ways, two men had only anonymous ways, twelve men had both social and anonymous ways, while eighteen of the 47 men had no way of making sexual contacts after awareness of seropositivity. Among these eighteen who did

Figure 3.

Number of the 47 men with different numbers of social ways (0-4) of making sexual contacts before and after awareness of the HIV infection

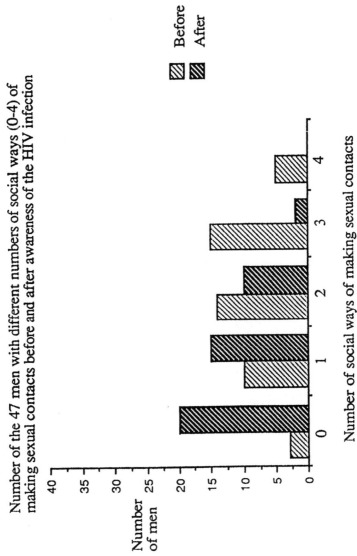

Figure 4.

Number of the 47 men with different numbers of anonymous ways (0-4) of making sexual contacts before and after awareness of the HIV infection

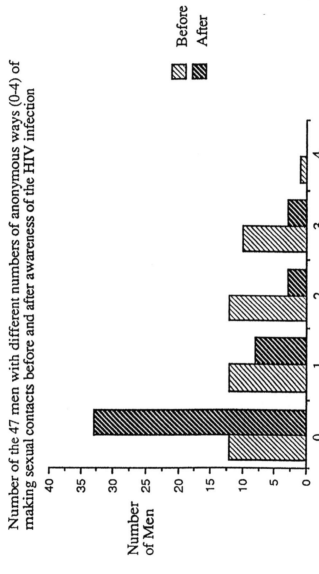

not take any new sexual contacts, eight were cohabiting and two had partners without cohabiting. Before awareness, 38 of the 47 men used to meet partners at bars or discotheques for gays, and after awareness only 21 did (p = 0.03) (Figure 5). Twenty-nine men used to make sexual contacts by "cruising" at gay meeting-places, i.e., parks, etc., before they were aware of the HIV infection, and afterwards only nine did (p = 0.01). All the other *ways* of making sexual contacts also decreased statistically significantly, i.e., in social life, by advertisements, at bars and discotheques, in saunas or video-clubs, at public toilets and on the telephone "contact line."

The frequency of *new sexual* contacts per year made in their habitual way also decreased after awareness of seropositivity. As a median the men made 24 (Range 1-108) new sexual contacts per year in their habitual way before they were aware of the seropositivity and only 1 (Range 1-24) contact afterwards (p < .001).

In the population different sexual contact patterns could be identified. Those men who continued to make new sexual contacts after HIV-diagnosis were characterized as being older (age over the mean, 39 years), having a partner or cohabiting with a friend, being a member of a gay organization or other organizations, being in contact with voluntary HIV organizations and in contact with a counsellor (odds ratios > 2) (Table 3).

Men who were members of some organization, a gay organization, or had contact with a voluntary HIV organization or a counsellor or men who experienced stress more often had both social and anonymous *ways* of making sexual contacts after awareness of their seropositivity (odds ratios > 2.5) (Table 4). White collar men more often had social *ways* of making sexual contacts (odds ratio = 2.7) (Table 4).

The social way was the most common *way* of making new sexual contacts after awareness of seropositivity for *all* white collar men but only for 78% of the blue collar men (p = 0.07), and for *all* those who were exclusively homosexual but only for 82% of the men who were not exclusively homosexual (p = 0.05).

In conclusion, those men who had ways to make sexual contacts and also made new contacts, after awareness of their seropositivity were more often members of an organization, members of a gay

Figure 5.

Number of the 47 men with different social and anonymous ways of making sexual contacts before and after awareness of the HIV infection

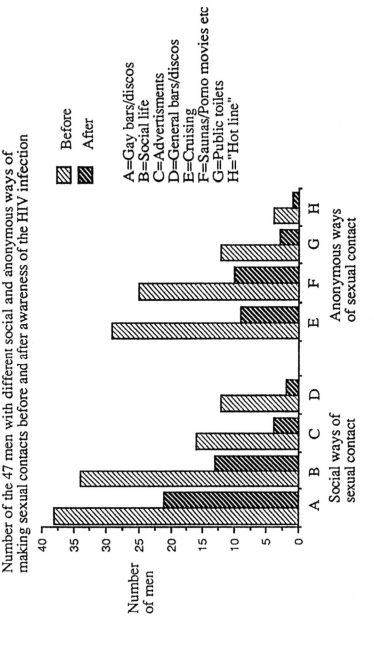

Before

After

A=Gay bars/discos
B=Social life
C=Advertisments
D=General bars/discos
E=Cruising
F=Saunas/Porno movies etc
G=Public toilets
H="Hot line"

Number of men

40
35
30
25
20
15
10
5
0

A B C D

Social ways of sexual contact

E F G H

Anonymous ways of sexual contact

organization, and had contact with a voluntary HIV organization or with a counsellor. According to a correlation analysis (Table 5) those men who were members of any organization more often had a partner or was living with a friend, had higher socio-economic status, were Swedish, and were members of a gay organization. Those men who had contact with a voluntary HIV organization more often were members of a gay organization or other organizations and they also experienced stress more often or were depressed. Men in contact with a counsellor also experienced more stress and they were more often members of a gay organization and had contact with a voluntary HIV organisation.

DISCUSSION

The objective of this study was to describe a representative city population of HIV antibody positive homosexual and bisexual men regarding their psychosocial situation, and to examine if and how awareness of their seropositivity and different psychosocial factors influenced the sexual contact pattern. After awareness of seropositivity there was a decrease in both the number of ways of making sexual contacts and the frequency of new sexual contacts. Men who had contact with HIV, gay or other organizations or a counsellor or experienced stress continued to make sexual contacts and also to a higher degree made new contacts after awareness of their seropositivity. Data also indicated that those men who had contact with a voluntary HIV organization were more depressed and experienced more stress.

The study population consists of almost all detected seropositive gay men without an AIDS diagnosis in Malmö. All detected gay men in Malmö are patients at the only clinic in the city that cares for persons seropositive for HIV. Only one person had contact with a private physician. An unknown number of men may have been tested outside Malmö. Most people, however, diagnosed with AIDS in Malmö during recent years have been known as seropositive patients at the Department of Infectious Diseases (Hansson H-B, 1991). This fact indicates that the study population is fairly representative of all HIV infected gay men in Malmö, both detected and undetected. This unique situation is explained by the fact that only one hospital department cares for HIV infected patients in Malmö and that quite a lot of people know of their HIV antibody status. The Swedish policy of HIV-antibody testing is somewhat different than in other countries. The subject's awareness of his/her HIV antibody status is seen as an important part in preventing the transmission of the infection. For people who may have exposed themselves to HIV infection, testing is mandatory in Sweden. It is easy to get access to a test in Sweden, many testing sites are available and the test is free of charge. Therefore, rather a lot of gay men have been tested.

In many non-HIV studies the non-participants have been shown to be a selected group of people with, for example, lower education, more social isolation and higher morbidity and mortality (Janzon, Hanson, Isacsson, Lindell & Steen, 1986). In the present work, however, a comparison between participants and non-participants showed only slight and no statistically significant differences. This indicates that the participants can be regarded as fairly representative of the whole study population. This fact implies that the associations found in this study are possibly not exaggerated.

Since the study population was rather small there was a loss of power in the statistical analysis. Therefore odds ratios had to attain levels above three in order to be statistically significant. However, since a rather high proportion of detected HIV infected gay men in Malmö were enrolled in the study, odds ratios higher than two were considered as interesting.

A marked change in sexual contact pattern after awareness of HIV infection was found in this study. It can be argued that factors like "social desirability" and "the need for approval" can bias the results, i.e., the interviewed men tend to answer in a socially desirable way to win approval from the interviewer (Crowne & Marlowe, 1960; Philips, 1973). However, all three interviewers have a good and lengthy knowledge of the patients and the gay community in Malmö. All participants are well-known patients at the Department of Infectious Diseases and they have been surveyed thoroughly, both psychosocially and medically. Experience from the clinical work at the Department and from work in a voluntary HIV support organization in Malmö supports the validity of the results in this study.

Results from other studies is in line with our findings. The sexual activity and the number of sexual partners decrease significantly after awareness of one's own seropositivity for HIV (van Griensven, Vroome, Tielman, Goudsmit & de Wolf, 1989). Even if a large number of *all* gay men, even those not seropositive for HIV, have changed their sexual contact pattern and sexual behavior because of the perceived risk of HIV, studies show that gay men seropositive for HIV have made the greatest changes. This is true especially for high risk sexual behaviors (McCusker, Stoddard, Mayer, Zapka, Morrison & Saltzman, 1988; Fox, Odaka, Brookmeyer & Polk, 1987).

To reduce or to have no sexual contacts after awareness of seropositivity for HIV can be seen as part of a general withdrawal from social life. Contacts with organizations are important sources of social support and can be regarded as psychosocial resources of importance when dealing with the demands of daily life and stressful life-events like becoming seropositive for HIV. The crisis that comes from the awareness of seropositivity can be difficult to handle (Weitz, 1989). It is then important to have access to good social support, i.e., persons to talk to and persons who can listen and give advice, comfort and support. To have good possibilities to make social, emotional and also sexual contacts and to make them last, can therefore reduce stress (Kiecolt-Glaser, 1988). Social isolation can also be hazardous for health in other ways. The lifestyle can become impoverished with more alcohol and tobacco consumption, more inadequate dietary habits, less physical activity, etc. (Hanson, Isacsson, Janzon & Lindell, 1989). Social isolation could also in a more direct way influence the course of the HIV infection resulting in earlier or more severe complications (Temoshok, 1988; Hanson, 1988).

The objectives of other studies have often been on sexual behavior, i.e., whether gay men practice receptive or insertive anal intercourse, or if a condom is used. In this study, however, the emphasis has been laid on the sexual contact patterns. Both social and sexual contacts between men can be made at different places such as gay discos, public toilets, in social life or through ''cruising'' in parks, etc. Some men have few ways of making sexual contact, while others have many. The different places or ways of making sexual contacts have in this study been divided into two groups, anonymous and social, where anonymous means contacts that do not have to include a social or emotional involvement. The two ways of making sexual contact are thus not equal regarding the possibilities of creating deeper social and emotional relations. This study does not reveal anything about the men's ways of having sex. We do not know if they are practicing safer sex or not. Our theory is that good psychosocial resources are helpful in breaking down social, emotional and also sexual isolation. One policy of decreasing the spread of HIV infection is to minimize the number of sexual contacts. However, a complementary view is that it is not the number of partners that is important, but the fashion in which people have sex, i.e., to practice safe sex. If psychosocial resources give the strength to break social isolation it may also help people in not having risky sex. A Swedish study on male homosexuals who were members of a gay organization supports this view. As many as 86% of these men had made risk reducing behavioral changes because of perceived risk of HIV (Håkansson, 1990).

Those men who continued to have ways of making sexual contacts, and also made new contacts after awareness of seropositivity, more often were members of gay, or other organizations, had contact with voluntary HIV organizations and counsellors. These men have a good availability of beneficial psychosocial resources. However, they also experienced stress and men who had contact with voluntary HIV organizations felt depressed. This can outline different coping styles. Men with better psychosocial resources know ways to get help and support and they have the possibility of working through their HIV problem in a more active way. This may explain why they were more stressed and depressed. Those men who changed their sexual contact pattern more, i.e., had the lowest amount of sexual contact ways and sexual contacts, had for example less contacts with voluntary HIV organizations and they were less stressed at the moment. These men may suppress their HIV problem. They might isolate themselves and be afraid of making new social and sexual contacts. This may jeopardize their health in the long run and their prognosis concerning the progression of the

HIV infection may be poorer (Hanson, 1988; Lovejoy & Sisson, 1989).

In our study membership of organizations, and especially of a gay organization, or contact with voluntary HIV organizations influenced the men's sexual contact patterns. The Michigan study on Chicago homosexual men referred to earlier in this paper did not show that gay social network affiliation was related to sexual behavioral change (Emmons, Joseph, Kessler, Wortman, Montgomery et al., 1986). One explanation to this, and the inconsistencies between the other studies described in the introduction of this paper, could be the fact that the results in these other studies are based on samples that are more or less selected and not representative of the general population of gay men. Reasons for this inconsistency could also be confounding factors which make the associations spurious and that the studies focus different items, i.e., sexual behavior and sexual contact patterns.

The theoretical framework of this study is the one of *social epidemiology*. Interest has been focused on sexual contact patterns and the importance of psychosocial resources, like membership and contacts with organizations and counsellors. Psychosocial resources give a person possibilities to handle demands and stressful situations in daily life. A good access to a psychosocial resource gives better chances to resist tendencies of social isolation. To have social, emotional and sexual contacts are important for an individual's self-esteem and psychological well-being. It is also essential for health, and might be of importance even for the progression of the HIV-infection. This will be studied in the prospective follow-up of these men.

REFERENCES

Carlsson, G. (1958). Social Mobility and Class Structure. Lund, Gleerups.

Cassel, J. (1976). The contribution of the social environment to host resistance. American Journal of Epidemiology, 104, 107-123.

CDC. Centers for Disease Control. (1986). Classification system for Human T-Lymphotropic Virus type III infections. Morbidity and Mortality Weekly Reports, 35, 334-38.

Chuang, H. T., Devins, G. M., Hunsley, J. & Gill, M. J. (1989). Psychosocial

Distress and Well-Being Among Gay and Bisexual Men With Human Immuno-
deficiency Virus Infection. American Journal of Psychiatry, 146, 876-880.
Coates, T. J., McKusick, L., Kuno, R. & Stites, D. P. (1989). Stress Reduction
Training Changed Number of Sexual Partners but Not Immunfunction in Men
with HIV. American Journal of Public Health, 79, 885-887.
Crowne, D. P., & Marlowe, D. (1960). The new scale of social desirability inde-
pendent of psychopathology. Journal of Consulting Psychology, 24, 349-354.
Ekstrand, M. L. & Coates, T. J. (1990). Maintainance of Safer Sexual Behaviors
and Predictors of Risky Sex: The San Francisco Men's Health Study. American
Journal of Public Health, 80, 973-977.
Emmons, C-A., Joseph, J. G., Kessler, R. C., Wortman, C. B., Montgomery, S.
B. & Ostrow, D. G. Psychosocial Predictors of Reported Behavior Change in
Homosexual Men at Risk for AIDS. (1986). Health Education Quarterly, 13,
331-345.
van Griensven, G. J. P., de Vroome, E. M. M., Tielman, R. A. P., Goudsmit, J.,
de Wolf, F., van der Noordaa, J. & Coutinho, R. A. (1989). Effect of Human
Immunodeficiency virus (HIV) antibody knowledge and high-risk sexual be-
havior with steady and nonsteady sexual partners among homosexual men.
American Journal of Epidemiology, 129, 596-603.
Groopman, J. E., Chen, F. W., Hope, J. A., Andrews, J. M., Swift, R. L., Benton,
C. V., Sullivan, J. L., Volberding, P. A., Sites, D. P., Landesman, S., Gold, J.,
Baker, L., Craven, D. & Boches, F. S. (1986). Serological characterization of
HTLV-III infection in AIDS and related disorders. Journal of Infectious Dis-
eases, 153, 736-741.
Groopman, J. E., Mayer, K. H., Sarngadharan, M., Ayotte, D., Finberg, R., Sliski,
A., Allan, J. D. & Gallo, R. (1985). Seroepidemiology of human T-lympho-
tropic virus type III among homosexual men with acquired immune deficiency
syndrome or generalized lymphadenopathy and among asymptomatic controls
in Boston. Annals of Internal Medicine, 102, 334-337.
Hanson, B.S. (1988). Social network, social support and health in elderly men. A
population study. Lund, Studentlitteratur, (Thesis).
Hanson, B. S., Isacsson, S-O., Janzon, L. & Lindell, S.-E. (1989). Social Network
and Social Support Influence Mortality in Elderly Men. The prospective population study of "Men born in 1914," Malmö, Sweden. American Journal of
Epidemiology, 130, 100-111.
Hanson, B.S., Isacsson, S-O., Janzon, L. & Lindell, S-E. (1990). Social support
and quitting smoking for good. Is there an association? Results from the population study "Men born in 1914," Malmö, Sweden. Addictive Behaviors, 15,
221-233.
Hanson, B.S. & Östergren, P-O. (1987). Different social network and social support characteristics, nervous problems and insomnia: Theoretical and methodological aspects on some results from the population study "Men born in
1914," Malmö, Sweden. Social Science of Medicine, 25, 849-59.
Hansson, H-B. (1991). Chief Medical Officer of Health in the city of Malmö.
Personal communication.

Hays, R. B., Kegeles, S. M., Coates, T. J. (1990). High HIV risk-taking among young gay men. AIDS, 4, 901-907.

Håkansson, C. (1990). Sexual Behavior in a Group of Swedish Homosexual Men. Acta Dermato-Venereologica (Stockholm), 70, 27-30.

Janzon, L., Hanson, B.S., Isacsson, S-O., Lindell, S-E. & Steen, B. (1986). Factors influencing participation in health surveys. Results from the prospective population study "Men born in 1914," in Malmö, Sweden. Journal of Epidemiology and Community Health, 40, 174-177.

Kiecolt-Glaser, J. K., Kennedy, S., Malkoff, S., Fisher, L., Speicher, C. E. & Glaser, R. (1988). Marital Discord and Immunity in Males. Psychosomatic Medicine, 50, 213-229.

Lovejoy, N. C. & Sissin, R. (1989). Psychoneuroimmunology and AIDS. Holistic Nursing Practice, 3, 1-15.

McCusker, J., Stoddard, A.M., Mayer, K.H., Zapka, J., Morrison, C. & Saltzman, S. P. (1988). Effects of HIV Antibody Test Knowledge on Subsequent Sexual Behaviors in a Cohort of Homosexually Active Men. American Journal of Public Health, 78, 462-467.

McKusick, L., Coates, T. J., Morin, S. F., Pollack, L. & Hoff, C. (1990). Longitudinal Predictors of Reductions in Unprotected Anal Intercourse among Gay Men in San Francisco: The AIDS Behavioral Research Project. American Journal of Public Health, 80, 978-983.

Ostrow, D. G., Monjan, A., Joseph, J., van Raden, M., Fox, R., Kingsley, L., Dudley, J. & Phair, J. (1989). HIV-Related Symptoms and Psychological Functioning in a Cohort of Homosexual Men. American Journal of Psychiatry, 146, 737-742.

Philips, D. L. (1973). Abandoning Method. San Francisco, California, Jossey-Bass.

Prieur, A. (1990). Gay Men: Reasons for Continued Practice of Unsafe Sex. AIDS Education and Prevention, 2, 110-117.

Reinherz, E. L. & Schlossman, S. F. (1980). The Differentiation and Function of Human T Lymphocytes. Cell, 19, 821-7.

Roffman, R. A., Gilmore, M. R., Gilchrist, L. D., Mathias, S. A. & Krueger, L. (1990). Continuing Unsafe Sex: Assessing the Need for AIDS Prevention Counseling. Public Health Reports, 105, 202-208.

Siegel, K., Krauss, B. J. (1991). Living with HIV Infection: Adaptive Tasks of Seropositive Gay Men. Journal of Health and Social Behavior, 32, 17-32.

Siegel, K., Mesagno, F. P., Chen, J-Y. & Christ, G. (1989). Factors distinguishing homosexual males practicing risky and safer sex. Social Science of Medicine, 28, 561-569.

Temoshok, L. (1988). Psychoimmunology and AIDS. Psychological Neuropsychiatric; and Substance Abuse Aspects of AIDS. In T. Peter Bridge et al., eds. New York, Raven Press.

Weitz, R. (1989). Uncertainty and the Lives of Persons with AIDS. Journal of Health and Social Behavior, 30, 270-281.

WHO. (1989). Reports from the World Health Organization.

Psychological Correlates
of Unprotected Intercourse
Among HIV-Positive Gay Men

Ulrich Clement, PhD

SUMMARY. Several studies address the problem of a 'relapse to unsafe sexual activity' among gay men, and discuss the danger of a new wave of HIV-infections. The present study analyzes psychological predictors of unprotected intercourse in a sample of 58 HIV-positive gay men. Fifteen persons out of this sample had at least occasionally unprotected anal or oral sex with ejaculation. This group displays a characteristic psychological profile. Compared to the control group, these men (1) are more depressive, (2) have a tendency to blame themselves for being infected, (3) use an avoiding coping style, and (4) trust more in external control by professionals than in internal control. A psychological interpretation is proposed that sexual behavior can be regarded as a distracting coping mechanism against depression that is used to deny the threatening reality of the infection. The need for psychotherapy for HIV-infected persons is emphasized.

Since 1984, several cohort studies have investigated changes in sexual behavior among gay men, as a response to the threat of AIDS. The Multicenter AIDS Cohort Study (MACS), the San Francisco Gay Men's Health Study, the Vancouver Lymphadenopathy Study and the New York Community Impact Project, and others have documented the feature of sexual behavior changes. These

Ulrich Clement is affiliated with Psychosomatic Hospital, University of Heidelberg, Thibautstrasse 2, 6900 Heidelberg, Germany.

Support for this research was provided by the Ministry of Science and Art, Baden-Wuerttemberg.

Lena Nilsson Schönnesson contributed the data of the Swedish subsample.

133

studies as well as comparable ones in Europe (Bochow, 1988; Dannecker, 1990; Pollack, 1990) conclude that gay and bisexual men have reduced the number of sex partners, confine largely to so-called 'safer sex' practices (i.e., no ejaculation in the mouth or anus), and increased use of condoms when having anal sex (for a review, see Becker & Joseph, 1988).

After these dramatic changes during the 1980s, the focus of interest at the beginning of the 1990s is shifting towards difficulties in maintaining 'safer sex' over a longer period of time. At the Sixth International Conference on AIDS in San Francisco, June 1990, several research groups reported about a 'relapse to unsafe sexual activity' in the gay community, and discussed the danger of a 'second wave' of infections.

The MACS (Kingsley, Bacellar, Zhou, Rinaldo, Chmiel, Detels, Saah, Van Raden, Ho, Armstrong, and Munoz, 1990) reports on a semiannual seroconversion rate of initially seronegative men. Between late 1984 and early 1988, the seroconversion rate dropped from 3.7 to 0.4/100 persons/semester, but increased again to 0.8 persons/semester within one year, i.e., until early 1989.

Willoughby, Schechter, Craib, McLeod, Douglas, Fay, Nitz, and O'Shaughnessy (1990) compared 51 men, who had seroconverted since 1985, to 189 men, who remained seronegative. The seroconverters were found to be younger, lower educated and to use drugs (amphetamines, cocaine, marijuana) more frequently than the non-converters. Another study (O'Reilly, Higgins, Galavotti, Sheridan, 1990), where a 6% 'relapse' rate within six months was reported, identified the following predictors of relapse: younger age, lack of a steady partner, low peer-support for condom use, and alcohol and drug use.

Adib, Joseph, and Ostrow (1990) found that gay men in monogamous relationships tended to practice more unsafe sex than singles. Among men without a steady partner, situational factors like alcohol or being 'turned on,' played a role in performing unsafe sex. Different studies have found a correlation between unsafe sex and use of drugs (Stall, McKusick, Wiley, Coates, and Ostrow, 1986; Ostrow, Beltran, Wesch, and Joseph, 1990). Different psychoactive substances (amphetamines: Harris, Sohlberg, and Livingston, 1990; Willoughby et al., 1990; alcohol: O'Reilly et al., 1990; Adib et al.,

1990; marijuana: Kegeles, Greenblatt, Cardenas, and Catania, 1990) were found to be associated with inconsistent 'safer sex.' It is important to note that this association cannot be explained by the substance alone, but attention has also to be paid to peer support and individual coping mechanisms to reduce distress. Most of these studies do not refer particularly to the HIV-status of the respondents.

Indirectly, they minimize the psychosexual impact of a positive HIV-status because they do not compare between subjects with positive, negative and unknown HIV-status. Sound knowledge about the sexual behavior of testpositive persons is essential for secondary prevention though. The purpose of this article is to illuminate and to achieve a better understanding of the psychological dynamics of unsafe sex among homosexual HIV-positive men. In other words: What are the reasons of some HIV-carriers to–at least occasionally–practice unprotected sex?

SAMPLE AND METHOD

In a German-Swedish[1] cooperative study, the psychological sequelae and the adaptation process of an HIV-infection are investigated. Fifty-eight self-identified gay men were in-depth interviewed; additionally they filled out questionnaires as to sexual behavior and attitudes, as well as various psychological parameters. The German subsample (N = 30) was made up of men from the Heidelberg area. Most of them were recruited from two HIV-clinics of the Medical School of the University of Heidelberg. The Swedish subsample (N = 28) was recruited in Stockholm through volunteer organizations. The criterion for being included in the study was to be diagnosed with HIV but not with AIDS. Subjects with neuropsychological symptoms were excluded from the study. Thus, the sample is not representative of homosexual HIV-carriers, since it is biased to those who are not physically impaired by the infection.

Among the 58 subjects, 15 of them reported that they had had unprotected oral and/or anal sex to ejaculation with a casual partner at least once after notification of their HIV-diagnosis. Eleven men had not had any casual partners after tested seropositive. Twenty-three had practiced consistently 'safer sex,' i.e., never had oral and/or anal sex to ejaculation after notification. Seven participants refused to respond to questions about their sexual behavior, and were excluded from the following analysis. The group who had unsafe sex (N = 15) is compared to the controls (N = 34) who have not taken the risk of infecting another person.

Twenty-nine percent of the sample (N = 49) were 30 years old or younger, 51% 31-40 years, and 20% older than 40 years (mean age: 38.8 years). Twenty-four percent were notified about their HIV-diagnosis less than one year, 26% between one and two years, and 50% more than two years (mean: 22.6 months).

ASSESSMENT

Personality: Personality traits were assessed by the Giessen-Test (Beckmann and Richter, 1982), a 40-item inventory forming six scales that are constructed on the basis of psychodynamic theory. The Giessen-Test is a reliable and an often used personality inventory in German clinical research.

Subjective infection theory: Four relevant subjective attributions of the HIV-infection were assessed: namely, 'internal' (the infected person blames himself for being infected), 'external' (the infected person blames someone else for being infected), 'chance' (no particular person is blamed) and 'fatalistic' (the infection is experienced as an expression of fate or a higher destiny).

Coping style: By coping *style*, we refer to an individual's cognitive and emotional way of coping with stressful events. Coping style, as conceptualized in this way, is more personality-dependent than situational. To assess coping styles, we used the Freiburg Coping List FKV (Muthny, 1986), an 80-items questionnaire making up 11 scales, that is derived from Lazarus' WCCL (Ways of Coping Check List).

Coping strategy: We developed a list of coping strategies, the Heidelberg HIV Coping List (HHCL), that consists of 28 items describing particular behaviors. The subjects were asked which behavior helps versus harms them in their living with HIV.

Attitudes towards changing sexual behavior: A 16-item-scale was used. This scale turned out to be psychometrically insufficient by its low internal consistency. A factor analysis yielded five factors. Based on these, five short (2-4 items) subscales were constructed: 'difficulties,' 'thoughtlessness,' 'positive reframing,' 'responsibility,' 'hedonism.'

Depressiveness and life satisfaction: 'Depressiveness' is a reliable (Cronbach's Alpha = .88) 6-item-subscale of the FKV. 'Life satisfaction' was assessed with the 'Fragebogen zur Lebenszufriedenheit' (Fahrenberg, Myrtek, Wilk, Kreutel, 1986). Subjects are coding their satisfaction versus dissatisfaction for eight areas of life.

The data are analyzed in two steps, first by comparing means of the relevant variables (t-tests) that are combined and alpha-adjusted in a second step by a multivariate model (stepwise discriminant analysis).

RESULTS

Personality Traits

The two groups clearly differ in one scale only, 'depressiveness,' the unsafe-sex group being more depressed (t = 2.2., p < .05).

'Subjective Infection Theory' (Attribution)

Table 1 shows a characteristic attribution profile of the unsafe-sex group. These men are significantly more concerned with internal attributions. They blamed themselves for the infection, in terms of psychic readiness, a tendency to have bad luck, etc. The external attribution is also marked in this group, but not on a significant level. However, it should be emphasized, that in both groups chance is the most common attribution. With respect to chance, the two groups are indifferent. The attribution profiles of both groups are predominated by the 'realistic' chance attribution. But there is a tendency among these men, who have problems in maintaining 'safer sex,' to also display a self-blaming attitude.

Table 1: Attribution * (` subjective infection theory`) by sexual behavior

	oral/anal sex with risk of infection (N = 15)	no risk of infection (N = 34)	t	p(t)
internal	1.71 (.35)	1.37 (.60)	2.00	.06
external	1.56 (.57)	1.33 (.32)		ns
fatalistic	1.27 (.32)	1.35 (.35)		ns
chance	2.18 (.58)	2.11 (.53)		ns

*   All scale ranges from 1 (not at all) to 3 (clearly); standard deviation in parentheses.

Coping Style

A main interest of the study concerns the way HIV-carriers cope with their traumatic diagnosis. The unsafe-sex group has a marked tendency to use an avoidant coping-style. Data also show that this group has a strong need of social support (Table 2). This could be interpreted as a tendency to be dependent upon others.

Coping Strategies

The unsafe-sex group codes 'talking about the future,' 'distraction from thinking about the infection,' 'going to psychotherapy,' and 'taking a cure' as being more helpful than the control group. In contrast, 'being often alone,' 'living exactly as before,' 'conscious and healthy alimentation,' 'reflecting on religious questions,' and 'continuing life without changes' are coded as being less helpful than by the control group (Table 3).

This puzzling feature contains two remarkable tendencies. First, the unsafe sex group rated behaviors that imply continuing life as it was before as being of little help (living exactly as before, continuing life without changes). Obviously they are less convinced that their life is worth living. This fits with the above mentioned depressive pattern.

Second, if we regard coping strategies in terms of internal versus external locus of control (Rotter, 1966), the better ratings of psychotherapy and medical treatment (external control), and the more negative ratings of 'healthy alimentation' (internal control) could be interpreted as a tendency to trust more in external control. Taken together with the more negative rating of 'being alone,' this tendency also fits with the coping-style of seeking social support.

The higher ratings of 'talking about the past' and 'distraction from thinking about the infection' in the unsafe-sex group could be a reflection of the coping style of avoidance.

Attitudes Towards Changing Behavior

As expected, changes in sexual behavior are rated differently between the two groups (Table 4). Corresponding to actual behav-

Table 2: Coping style* by sexual behavior

	oral/anal sex with risk of infection (N = 15)	no risk of infection (N = 34)	t	p(t)
avoidance/ wishful thinking	3.30 (1.22)	2.28 (.94)	3.14	.01
seeking for social support	3.31 (.66)	2.79 (.59)	2.74	.01

* Scale range from 1 (not at all) to 5 (very much); standard deviation in parentheses.

ior, the subjects of the unsafe-sex group in contrast to the control group expressed more difficulties and a slightly (not significantly) more thoughtless and less responsible attitude.

Depressiveness and Life Satisfaction

The participants who made up the unsafe-sex group are markedly more depressive and less satisfied with several aspects of life (Table 5) than the others. It is surprising that satisfaction with sexual life does not differ between the two groups.

Multivariate Analysis of the Predictor Variables

The above presented successive bivariate analyses have the advantage that particular aspects of the psychological feature can be focused upon separately. The statistical problem is, however, that the predictors are intercorrelated. Thus, the significance level is lower, and the predictive power of the whole set of significant parameters is overestimated.

These problems are taken into consideration when a stepwise discriminant analysis is calculated. The stepwise discriminant analysis includes the relevant predictors by their additional explanation of variance. Sexual behavior (unsafe sex versus control group) is here the criterion variable.

The first discriminant analysis includes the personality scales of the Giessen-Test, the subjective infection theory and coping-style. Table 6 shows that 'avoidance' and 'withdrawal' explain 24% of the criterion variance. Another 6% are explained by 'depressiveness.' These three predictors form a consistent depressive-avoidant pattern.

The second discriminant analysis includes the coping strategies that differed significantly between the two groups (Table 7). Five relatively diverse strategies determine over 50% of the variance: 'going to psychotherapy,' 'often being alone,' 'living as before,' 'reflecting on religious questions,' and 'taking a cure.'

The third stepwise discriminant analysis includes the attitudes towards sexual behavior change (Table 8). Surprisingly, these attitudes predict only 18%.

Table 3: Coping strategies * by sexual behavior

	oral/anal sex with risk of infection (N = 15)	no risk of infection (N = 34)	t	p(t)
Talking about the past	4.14 (.86)	3.53 (.88)	2.18	.05
often being alone	2.14 (1.17)	2.91 (1.09)	2.14	.05
distraction from thinking about the infection	3.92 (.83)	3.44 (.76)	1.96	.05
living exactly as before	3.07 (1.33)	4.00 (1.16)	2.39	.05
conscious and healthy alimentation	4.07 (.73)	4.47 (.76)	1.64	.10

reflecting on religious questions	2.71 (1.13)	3.31 (.82)	2.01	.05
continuing my life without changes	2.93 (1.44)	3.75 (1.14)	2.01	.05
going to psychotherapy	4.64 (.63)	3.94 (.76)	3.03	.01
taking a cure	4.29 (.83)	3.69 (.56)	2.49	.05

* Scale range: 1 (hurts a lot), 2 (hurts partly), 3 (neither hurts nor helps), 4 (helps partly), 5 (helps a lot); standard deviation in parentheses

Table 4: Attitudes towards changing sexual behavior* by sexual behavior

	oral/anal sex with risk of infection (N = 15)	no risk of infection (N = 34)	t	p(t)
difficulties	2.07 (.55)	1.63 (.49)	2.73	.01
responsibility	2.08 (.61)	2.38 (.49)	1.71	.10
thoughtlessness	1.38 (.46)	1.13 (.28)	1.88	.10

* Scale range 1 (not at all) to 3 (clearly); standard deviation in parentheses

In summary, the coping-strategies yielded the best prediction of unsafe sexual behavior. If 'depressiveness' is included, 64% of the criterion variance can be determined by the following four predictors: depressive feelings and the coping strategies 'psychotherapy,' 'not reading about AIDS,' and 'not being alone' (Table 9). The discriminant functions of these four parameters adequately predict 13/14 of the unsafe-sex group and 30/32 of the control group, i.e., 93.5%.

DISCUSSION

Among the 15 HIV-positive gay men who reported occasionally practicing unprotected oral or anal sex, a distinct psychological profile can be identified. Based upon a depressive personality, these men have a tendency to blame themselves (in terms of their character or their psychic readiness) for being infected. They also display an avoiding coping-style, i.e., they tend to deny the implications of the diagnosis (obviously, unprotected sex is a symptom of denial) by indulging into wishful thinking and to withdraw from social contacts. As a consequence of this restricted confrontation with their situation, they make use of coping-strategies that rely on professional help and on avoidance of reflecting upon the implications of their infection. This coping pattern results in depressive feelings and a general dissatisfaction with various aspects of life.

For an interpretation of the psychological dynamics of unprotected intercourse, I propose to begin with the internal attribution of the HIV-infection. In the case of a sexually transmitted HIV-infection, it would seem evident that the person's past sexual life, and possibly his gay identity, is blamed for the actual situation. Janoff-Bulman (1977) has introduced the terms *characterological self-blame* and *behavioral self-blame*. She found in her studies with accident victims, that those who blame a particular and relatively limited behavior as being responsible for the traumatic event (behavioral self-blame) will get along better with it than those who blame their whole person and their character (characterological self-blame).

In the case of an HIV-infection that has been transmitted sexually, it could be argued that characterological self-blame in terms of

Table 5: Depressive feelings and dissatisfaction by sexual behavior*

	oral/anal sex with risk of infection (N = 15)	no risk of infection (N = 34)	t	p(t)
depressive feelings**	3.55 (.99)	2.46 (.91)	3.70	.001
dissatisfaction***				
.....with work	4.69 (2.13)	3.27 (1.91)	2.19	.05

.....with leisure time	3.87 (1.55)	2.88 (1.43)	2.16	.05
.....with partner situation	4.75 (2.25)	2.75 (2.09)	2.30	.05
.....with myself	3.93 (1.49)	3.06 (1.31)	2.02	.05

*   Standard deviation in parentheses
**   Scale range: 1 (not at all) to 5 (very much)
***   Scale range: 1 (very satisfied) to 7 (very dissatisfied)
         4 (neither satisfied nor dissatisfied)

Table 6: Stepwise discriminant analysis: Prediction of sexual behavior from personality traits, attribution, and coping-style

Variable	partial r^2	F	p(F)	Wilks` Lambda	p (Lambda)	ASCC*	p(ASCC)
1 avoidance/ wishful thinking	.18	9.8	.003	.82	.003	.18	.003
2 withdrawal	.08	4.0	.05	.75	.002	.24	.002
3 depressivity	.08	3.8	.05	.69	.001	.31	.001

* Average squared canonical correlation

Table 7: Stepwise discriminant analysis: Prediction of sexual behavior from coping strategies

Variable	partial r^2	F	p(F)	Wilks' Lambda	p (Lambda)	ASCC*	p(ASCC)
1 Psychotherapy	.17	9.2	.004	.83	.004	.17	.004
2 often being alone	.14	7.1	.010	.71	.0006	.29	.0006
3 living as before	.09	4.6	.04	.64	.0003	.36	.0003
4 reflecting on religious questions	.12	5.6	.02	.56	.0001	.44	.0001
5 taking a cure	.09	4.1	.05	.51	.0001	.49	.0001

* Average squared canonical correlation

Table 8: Stepwise discriminant analysis: Prediction of sexual behavior from coping strategies

Variable	partial r^2	F	p(F)	Wilks` Lambda	p (Lambda)	ASCC*	p(ASCC)
1 difficulties	.11	5.3	.03	.89	.03	.11	.03
2 thoughtlessness	.08	3.7	.06	.82	.01	.18	.01

* Average squared canonical correlation

homosexual identity and sexual life-style will be at focus. In other words, this characterological self-blame seems connected with an internalized homophobia.

If sexual identity is to be blamed, the respective person will hide his HIV-diagnosis even more (avoiding coping-style), will deny it and withdraw from social exchange, resulting in depressiveness and pessimism about the future. This might give an explanation to the clinical observation that these individuals are not in touch with peer support, feel less responsibility towards the gay community not to further transmit the infection, have less access to AIDS prevention campaigns and, which is more important, do not feel personally addressed by the new community standard of 'safer sex.'

The results of the discriminant analysis of the coping-strategies that predict unprotected sexual behavior complete this feature: HIV-infected men who are less inclined to confront themselves with their situation (i.e., rating 'being alone' and 'being concerned about religious questions' as harmful), and who are pessimistic with respect to their future life up to now (rating 'continuing life as it was' as harmful) and have a strong need for professional help (rating psychotherapy and medical treatment as helpful) are apt to practice unsafe sex. Their individual helplessness and their need for professional help, especially psychotherapy, is important to note.

The relevant psychological process that might explain unsafe sexual behavior on the background of this depressive-avoidant feature is the depression-reducing function of sexuality. A sexual encounter can give a relief from depression and anxiety at least for a moment. Sexual behavior can be a distracting coping mechanism that helps to forget the threatening reality for a moment. The more threatening this reality is, the less energy is left for negotiating about 'safer sex.'

AIDS prevention must be much more aware of the psychological and psychosexual situation of the more isolated and less integrated persons with HIV/AIDS. Individual and group psychotherapy for them should become an integrated part of AIDS prevention.

Table 9: Stepwise discriminant analysis: Prediction of sexual behavior from depressive feelings and coping strategies

Variable	partial r^2	F	p(F)	Wilks Lambda	p (Lambda)	ASCC*	p(ASCC)
1 depressive feelings	.24	13.5	.0007	.76	.0007	.24	.0007
2 psychotherapy	.26	14.1	.0005	.56	.0001	.44	.0001
3 reading about AIDS	.26	13.9	.0006	.42	.0001	.58	.0001
4 often being alone	.14	6.4	.02	.36	.0001	.64	.0001

Classification by discriminative functions

	Prediction	
	risk of infection	no risk of infection
risk of infection	13	2
no risk of infection	1	30
total	14	32
rate of mistakes	7.1%	6.3%

* Average squared canonical correlation

153

NOTE

1. Principal investigator of the Swedish project is Lena Nilsson Schönnesson.

REFERENCES

Adib, M., Joseph, J., Ostrow, D. (1990): Relapse in safer sexual practices among homosexual men: Two year follow-up from the Chicago-MACS. Sixth International Conference on AIDS, San Francisco California, USA, June 20-24, 1990, F.C. 724

Becker, M.H., Joseph, J.G. (1988): AIDS and behavioral change to reduce risk: A review. American Journal of Public Health 78:394-410

Beckmann, D., Richter, H.E. (1972): Der Giessen-Test. Bern: Huber

Bochow, M. (1988) Wie leben schwule Männer heute? Bericht über eine Befragung im Auftrag der Deutschen AIDS-Hilfe. AIDS-Forum D.A.H., Band II, Berlin

Dannecker, M. (1990): Homosexuelle Männer und AIDS–Eine sexualwissenschaftliche Studie zu Sexualverhalten und Lebensstil. Schriftenreihe des Bundesministers für Jugend, Familie, Frauen und Gesundheit, Band 252. Stuttgart: Kohlhammer

Fahrenberg, J., Myrtek, M., Wilk, D., Kreutel, K. (1986): Multimodale Erfassung der Lebenszufriedenheit: Eine Untersuchung an Herz-Kreislauf-Patienten. Psychotherapie medizinische Psychologie 36:347-354

Harris, N., Sohlberg, E., Livingston, G. (1990): HIV spread among intravenous drug users (IVDUs) in King County, Washington. Sixth International Conference on AIDS, San Francisco California, USA, June 20-24, 1990, F.C. 564

Janoff-Bulmann, R. (1977) Characterological versus behavioral self-blame: Inquiries into depression and rape. Journal of Personality and Social Psychology 37:1798-1809

Kegeles, S., Greenblatt, R., Cardenas, C., Catania, J., Ontiveros, T., Coates, T.J. (1990): How do hispanic and white adolescent women differ in sexual risk behavior and in their antecendants? Sixth International Conference on AIDS, San Francisco California, USA, June 20-24, 1990, F.C. 733

Kingsley, L.A., Bacellar, H., Zhou, S., Rinaldo, C., Chmiel, J., Detels, R., Saah, H., Van Raden, M., Ho, M., Armstrong, J., Munoz, A. (1990): Temporal trends in seroconversion. A report from the Multicenter AIDS Cohort Study (MACS). Sixth International Conference on AIDS, San Francisco California, USA, June 20-24, 1990, F.C. 550

Muthny, F.A. (1986): Freiburger Fragebogen zur Krankheitsverar-beitung. Manuscript, version 6/1986

O'Reilly, K.R., Higgins, D.L., Galavotti, C., Sheridan, J. (1990): Relapse from safer sex among homosexual men: Evidence from four cohorts in the AIDS community demonstration projects. Sixth International Conference on AIDS, San Francisco California, USA, June 20-24, 1990, F.C. 717

Ostrow, D., Beltran, E., Wesch, J., Joseph, J. (1990): Recreational drug use and homosexual behavior: The role of volatile nitrites ('poppers') in explaining the association. Sixth International Conference on AIDS, San Francisco California, USA, June 20-24, 1990, F.C. 726

Pollack, M. (1990): Homosexuelle Lebenswelten im Zeichen von AIDS. Soziologie der Epidemie in Frankreich. Ergebnisse sozialwissen-schaftlicher AIDS-Forschung 4. edition sigma: Berlin

Rotter, J.B. (1966) Generalized expectancies for internal versus external control of reinforcement. Psychological Monographs 80:1-28

Stall, R., McKusick, L., Wiley, J., Coates, T.J., Ostrow, D.G. (1986): Alcohol and drug use during sexual activity and compliance with safe sex guidelines for AIDS: The AIDS Behavioral Research Project. Health Education Quarterly 13:359-371

Willoughby, B.C., Schechter, M.T., Craib, K.J.B., McLeod, W.A., Douglas, B., Fay, S., Nitz, R., O'Shaughnessy, M. (1990): Characteristics of recent seroconverters in a cohort of homosexual men: Who are the prevention failures? Sixth International Conference on AIDS, San Francisco California, USA, June 20-24, 1990, F.C. 45

Dead-End or Turning Point:
On Homosexuality and Coping with HIV

Sven-Axel Månsson, PhD

SUMMARY. The main question asked in this paper is: how do the more long-term survival strategies among HIV-positive homosexual men vary with the notion of themselves as homosexuals? This question is discussed in the light of two case studies that were selected from a sample of 16 HIV-positive homosexual men in a study on homosexuality and HIV performed by the author in Sweden during 1987-88. The two cases illustrate the complex interaction between a person's sexual orientation identity and his reactions to becoming HIV-positive, both in a short and long-term perspective. The conclusion of the qualitative analysis is that to some, being HIV-positive is the beginning of a dynamic personal development, while in others it causes a strong homophobic reaction, which is closely connected with the person's aversion to regarding himself as homosexual.

INTRODUCTION

To be diagnosed with HIV is a revolutionizing event in most respects. This is clearly manifested in the interviews I have conducted with 16 HIV-positive homosexual men (Månsson and Hilte, 1990). These men's experiences of the HIV-infection and their adaptation to it present many points of similarities, but at the same time there are considerable individual differences.

The course of the process can be divided into at least two phases, i.e., the acute phase of crisis and the phase of adaptation. The HIV-positive is confronted with various developmental tasks depending

Sven-Axel Månsson is Professor of Social Work, University of Gothenburg, Spranjeullsgaten 23, 411 23 Gothenburg, Sweden.

on which phase he is in. In the first one, he is faced with the task of relating, on an emotional as well as on a cognitive level, to the fact that he has become infected. In the second one, the individual is faced with the task of incorporating his changed living conditions with his everyday life and of trying to bring about a meaningful existence despite the limitations which the disease entails.

Also depending on which phase the men are in, some factors seem to be more outstanding than others when reaction patterns and adaptation strategies are determined. The basic element of the acute phase of crisis is on one hand the anxiety for stigmatization and becoming an outcast (i.e., the threat against one's social existence), on the other the anxiety for disease and death (i.e., the threat against one's human existence) (Nilsson Schönnesson, 1991). The sources of this anxiety are to be found in the social surroundings as well as within the individual himself and also in the interplay of these two factors. The social and cultural ideas attached to the disease are of great importance to the men's reaction patterns. Even at an early stage AIDS was described as a plague-like disease, the victims of which had largely themselves to blame for what had happened to them. Thus the interpretation of the men's strong emotional reactions cannot solely be made in the light of the biological characteristics of the disease. The way in which the disease is construed in the social surroundings and in the minds of people is of vital importance to the men's reactions. The HIV-diagnosis evokes strong feelings of shame and self-contempt at the same time as it calls up earlier, often unsolved, problems and conflicts connected with the person's homosexual actions and experiences.

In a processual perspective, the acute phase of crisis is followed by the individual's long-term adaptation to an existence as an HIV-positive. During this second phase the individual works through his experience of the disease, little by little reaching a stage where his mental suffering can be kept under control for longer periods. We might say that the emotional waves are "levelled out" to some extent and that more and more room is provided for a constructive way of functioning. However, it sometimes happens that the acute crisis turns into a more "chronic crisis" which means that the individual remains in a state characterized by regression, denial and emotional chaos. Even if this is rather exceptional, the dominant pattern being that the individual gradually advances and makes a move towards an acceptance of the thought of having to live with what has occurred, it has to be pointed out that the HIV-diagnosis involves a continuous and life-long adaptation process, where the psychological well-being has to be reclaimed and regained, over and over again.

The individual's attitude towards homosexuality and the homosexual form of life he has chosen is of great significance to his adaptation. One working hypothesis of the study was–in brief–that the more the men could agree with themselves about their sexual orientation and form of life, the more constructive and functional survival strategies concerning HIV were worked out and vice versa.

In a short-time perspective this hypothesis did not seem to be correct since in the acute phase of crisis it was not only the ambivalent men who repudiated their homosexual actions. Also among those men who earlier, more or less frankly, had manifested their homosexuality to the world around them, the traumatic diagnosis caused a dramatic redefinition in this respect. Strong and conflicting feelings of chaos, confusion and denial characterized the men's reactions in this phase. So the question was: what could be expected in a later phase, when these strong and conflicting feelings had "levelled out" concurrently with the men's gradual acceptance of having to live with the disease. What did the more long-term survival strategies look like? How did these strategies vary with the men's notion of themselves as homosexuals? And in what way did this notion obstruct or facilitate the men's long-term adaptation to a life as an HIV-positive?

DEVELOPMENT, ADAPTATION AND THE HOMOSEXUAL FORM OF LIFE

Generally, a traumatic crisis is not only to be regarded as a serious disturbing factor but also as a challenge. The crisis can be a call for a new way of acting. The challenge it provokes may produce new lines of action increasing the individual's adaptability and even improving his mental force. In this respect there are no sharp boundaries between traumatic crises and what is called developmental crises. A developmental crisis is a state which can be caused "by such external events which can be regarded as belonging to normal life but which nevertheless become too much for the individual in certain cases: to have children, to go out to work after being a housewife, to retire, etc." (Cullberg, 1984, p. 28). Certain experiences and developmental stages challenge the individual's inner experiences and his self-image. It is part of our life and of the human process of maturity to feel uncertain, worried, filled with anguish, doubting one's worth and the meaning of life, at times during rather long periods. The individual, however, often interprets this as symptoms of illness. Among other things the strict standards of normality in society contribute to this.

The anxiety connected with sexual orientation identity formation has been particularly evident to the men in the study. In a society as ours where there is no generally recognized homosexual form of life, the experience of not being sufficiently "normal" and of being an outcast has permeated the individual process of maturity. It has been a process filled with constant reconsideration, painful developmental leaps and sudden changes from intimacy to loneliness, from action to longing, from growth to stagnation. It is in this dynamic process these men are suddenly informed that they are ill. The traumatic experience–becoming HIV-positive–further disrupts their lives.

For some of them this occurs during a period of relative harmony, when the individual has learned to live with the sudden changes and has perhaps even succeeded in creating a feeling of balance between how he perceives himself and how he appears before the world.

For others, the infection interferes in a situation dominated by strong feelings of conflict as regards their own homosexuality, where their form of life might change between periods of full expression of their homosexuality and periods of celibacy interspersed with denunciation and feelings of shame and disgust. Still others have ordered their lives according to traditional heterosexual principles including marriage and having a family, while at the same time leading a secret homosexual life.

Form of Life and Scope of Action

Naturally, the forms of life mentioned above allow for different scopes of action for the strategies dealing with HIV. By scope of action I here mean, among other things, the individual's access to a social network which can support the process of adaptation. For example, a man who has chosen to conceal, in all essentials, his homosexual orientation and actions from the world around him will have difficulties in talking to other people about his condition. From his point of view, talking about HIV will be the same as talking about his homosexuality. The experience becomes a dramatic challenge of the entire form of life he has acquired. He suddenly realizes that he is all alone in the world. In the environment where he probably was infected there is nobody to turn to–nobody he wants to turn to. Besides, the very "arrangement" is based upon anonymous contacts. In the other environment, the one he has "protected" from knowing about the life he has led, there might be nobody he dares to confide in. The mere thought of surveying the consequences of his distress may seem too much for him in such a situation. To these individuals the process of adaptation will become prolonged and extremely painful.

TWO CASES

In order to demonstrate the different scopes of action for dealing with HIV, I have selected two cases from the 16 in the study. The reason for selecting these two is that they clearly demonstrate the two most common patterns found in the study, regarding the impact of sexual orientation identity on the process of adaptation to HIV.

This is Eric's story:

Looking back it's rather ironical. Seven years ago I was going to get married. I was happy. Now everything is different. Actually, I've got nothing to look forward to any longer. To be sure, my job still means a lot but on the other hand I have worked so much in my life . . . Besides, I'm mentally handicapped, because I know what I'm affected by. I can't help thinking about it for a minute, not even for a second. You can't go in for anything fully; a new job is not to be thought of. In that case you have to feel all right, at least in your brain.

It's awfully tragic being HIV-positive; a life without a future. I've felt like that all the time and I still do after three years. The future is in the past. At the same time I get these feelings now and then, although I try to resist them, that if I can manage another two years, put up with it, there might be some sort of effective medicines, even a vaccine that makes it possible for me to meet a girl and get married and perhaps have children. I don't often think like that but it has happened. There is one thing I've learned. There is nothing to be afraid of any more. Being HIV-positive is worse than anything. Nothing can scare you after that. And if I can cope it might be good to know that I don't have to be scared anymore. But even if I realize this, I suppose the truth is that it will never be of any use to me.

My life has come to a standstill and it has been like that for nearly three years. It's an odd feeling. I used to be very busy, always on the go. I was a successful salesman, travelling a lot, both at home and abroad. And it has been like that from the very moment I left home in the late 60s.

I grew up in a little village. My parents died when I was a teenager. I was much younger than my brothers and sisters and somehow my parents were always old. Country life was dull and I longed for living in town. After senior high school I went to the University of Gothenburg. Life there seemed smart to me. My studies were successful. I practised in New York for one year and learned properly how to push myself forward. And when I came home everything went smoothly and my career was terrific.

In the late 70s I had a lasting relationship with a wonderful girl. She had children from a previous relationship. We lived together and got on well. Now and then I had been going out with men, mostly when I was travelling abroad. It was quite the thing then, trying it out. I didn't take it so seriously. But the problem was that I seldom or never wanted to make love to her. I excused myself by saying that I had overworked myself but in the end that didn't sound very convincing. She began to realize what was the matter with me and after some time we split up. This was in the early 80s and I was filled with despair because what I wanted was a family and that other thing meant nothing. I didn't want to live as a gay–lacking a career, a family, children, a mother-in-law, in fact everything you are lacking when you are a full-time gay. Gays are so garrulous and shallow in their relations. The only thing that is important is what will happen next Saturday, and the next . . . That's not a life, I had discovered that. I did not want to live like that.

When I was informed that I was infected it came like a bombshell and I haven't got over it yet. My first thought was, "Don't tell anybody about this because they don't know very much about the disease. Don't show anything. Go to work as usual, behave as if nothing had happened." The feelings of shame, the fear! The fear of being disclosed, the fear of death. I kept to myself, walking about like a zombie for six months, completely self-absorbed. I went to work in order to avoid thinking; I worked till I was so tired that I wasn't able to think over all the consequences. I didn't talk to anybody about what had happened except my doctor, but he just gave me an encouraging pat on the back and said, "Live as you always have; that's the only thing to do."

In the end I suppose he understood that I was really feeling bad, so he advised me to join one of those support groups for HIV-positives initiated by the RFSL (the National Swedish Association for Sexual Equality). I needed badly to talk to someone so I went there. But that was indeed a mistake; I can see that now. Having been in that group for a while I felt even worse. Everything was focused on being gay. They spoke more about how oppressed gays had been at all times than about being HIV-positive. It was about "gays' lib" all the time. It was a complete nonsense. Not only that, we had to stand there cuddling each other, it was just disgusting, I didn't feel like being that intimate. I wanted them to answer my questions about HIV, but that didn't happen. The leaders were amateurs, they didn't know how to organize these things. Actually, it was horrible. One chap would sit there saying, "Oh, to me it has almost been a

good thing having HIV . . . and so on." Another one had had a
sickness pension for the past ten years and was still making trips to
the Arab countries. I was depressed as I myself had been infected
more or less in the same way. "Have I really been living like
them?" I thought. "No, I haven't, except for short periods when I
have been on holiday or travelling around in my job. And after all,
it's irrelevant now how I have lived."

I am HIV-positive and I've been infected in the usual way, I
don't deny that. But why harp about that? It was the only thing
they did in that group; talking about their way of life and their
identity, again and again. It was like some kind of hysteria and it
definitely gave me no comfort. I had already dissociated myself
from everything connected with homosexuality. But how should I
live now? How shall I cope with my social life as HIV-positive?
But the leaders were amateurs and I suppose they didn't know how
to handle it. It was depressing and I was feeling more and more
gloomy.

And I didn't get much help at the clinic either. It didn't seem to
me that the doctors took me seriously. If only there had been a real
doctor there who had been able to tell me how the disease would
affect me. But no!

After that I have decided to cope with this all by myself from
now on because it makes no difference if I tell somebody about it.
Not even my friends. Some time ago I told two friends of mine,
they are, you know, over-sympathetic, quite as the doctors . . . ,
"that doesn't make you ill if you don't want to, . . . you shouldn't
make so much fuss about it" and so on. Then I told two other
friends who are gays. But I shouldn't have done that. They didn't
react at all. Or, to be more correct, one of them, he is so sad . . .
"how are you feeling now? . . . how are you?" If you aren't depressed before, you will be. My youngest sister knows it, too. I
should never have told her, because she is almost more grieved
over it than I am. Her whole life has been destroyed. Is he going to
die now? she keeps thinking. You can put up with your own suffering, but others' too, that's difficult.

Now almost three years have passed and I'm still thinking,
"What's happened actually? How will it affect my life?" These
thoughts are painful. The first year I was most afraid of dying; that

was in fact the easiest thing to get over. I have had many pals who have died young in accidents and of diseases. I am over forty now and have had an eventful and varied life, so death doesn't frighten me. But now it's worse. Looking for symptoms! . . . The first sign of being ill. It's a terrible way of tormenting oneself. Every little complaint . . ."now I'm in for it!" I had a sore throat a week ago. I was absolutely paralyzed with fear and couldn't sleep at night.

It was then I lost my head entirely. I had drunk a bottle of wine as I couldn't sleep that night. In the morning I went to the clinic and blew up at the doctor. I just poured out all my miseries. "I think it's a crying shame," I said. "We've put a whole billion kronor in Sweden in this bloody AIDS epidemic. Where the hell is that money?". . . Everybody is to be informed, but the poor devils who are really in trouble, what kind of help have they got? Oh yes, they send you to Noah's Ark, a voluntary organization with a lot of half-time amateurs. Do you want me to go there and ask for help, a place where I can see AIDS and HIV written on everything and where there are a lot of people, so-called volunteers, prying about. How the devil shall I bring myself to go to them? I've worked and supported myself since I was 24 and I've paid taxes like hell. So why shouldn't I be helped by this hospital now that this has happened to me? How the devil do you think a group of volunteers should be able to help me in this jam. Besides, you may very well ask what kind of people are willing to help sick people of their own free will, without being paid. This is certainly not the case if you take a look at any other diseases, but AIDS . . . that's just terrific, because it's an in-thing while it lasts. I suppose people like that have got lost in life; they have been drifting around a lot and now they are thinking, "We'll start helping people with AIDS, you may get a kick out of it." I was terribly angry and I said to him, "Now I have to find a psychologist because I need to talk."–"Well," he began, there is one at the clinic here and then there are a few in town, they are gays, so they can . . ."–"I don't want any bloody gay," I shouted, "they are like water, . . . I need to talk. Haven't you got any good psychologists here. Surely, sick people must have been admitted to this hospital at all times, people with cancer and other things. There must be somebody here who knows something about how damned lousy I feel!"

OK, I calmed down in the end but the help I needed I never got. I got in touch with a psychologist, it's true, but she was also on about that gay talk, at first. And I told her I was absolutely uninterested in this matter. On the whole I have lost all interest in everything connected with sex and, what is worse, I have lost all interest in social life in general.

In Eric's account there are several themes we recognize from the acute phase of crisis: shock reaction, withdrawal, feelings of shame, fear, anger. When I saw him three years later, he still had great difficulties in accepting, let alone tolerating, the fact of the HIV-infection. He would not acknowledge the doctors' medical expertise. They cannot explain the disease. In his mind there was probably a hope that they–through their incompetence–had actually made a wrong diagnosis. He was offended at the way he had been treated within the nursing system, where the responsibility for the care, in his opinion, had been shifted on to amateurs, whose competence and motives he strongly doubted.

Eric's reactions against being regarded and treated as a homosexual is a main thread all through his story. For a long time he had been realizing that the homosexual life means nothing to him. The price was too high: no family, no children. In the end, however, he has paid a higher price than he would have suspected. He never says so himself, but we can read between the lines. But now it is enough. From now on he wants to be treated as an ordinary human being. The only problem is that the surrounding world insists that he should be treated as the "gay" he does not want to be. The doctors recommend him to try the RFSL's support group for HIV-positive homosexual men. He goes to this group because he needs somebody to share his experiences with. But he soon finds out that he has to confess to a homosexual identity to get any help there. "Everything was focused on being gay . . . (they were) talking about their way of life and their identity, again and again. It was like some kind of hysteria and it definitely gave me no comfort."

One might say that this experience caused a strong homophobic reaction in Eric. Homophobia is usually defined as "the irrational fear or intolerance of homosexuality" (Lehne, 1989, p. 416). The phenomenon may comprise whole communities or groups in the community as well as individuals. The main features of the social homophobia are prejudices and stereotyped conceptions of homosexuality and an underlying fear of becoming "infected" by this sexual "perversion." American studies of homophobia among men supports the thought that homophobia serves as a motivation, a driving force, in their ambition to maintain a distinct heterosexual identity. Even those men who have had sex with other men and who manifest clear homophobic attitudes and reactions in various studies often have a highly traditional outlook on gender roles and sexual preference (Lehne, 1989, p. 423). Moreover, many of these men do not regard their sexual contacts with other men as an expression of homosexuality. Being stigmatized as a homosexual threatens their existence and consequently these individuals tend to deprecate homosexuality and homosexuals–often more intensely and aggressively than other people do–with a view to controlling their own and other people's definition of their sexual preferences.

Eric's reactions to the meeting with the support group might be interpreted as an expression of such an experience of threat. As he says himself, "I had already dissociated myself from everything connected with homosexuality." Closely connected with the aggression he feels towards the homosexuals in the support group are also the bitterness and the desperation at not getting any support, because he does not belong to "the chosen ones." There is no alternative for a man like him; that is how he feels. "How am I now to live? How shall I manage living as an HIV-positive?" His own answer to these questions is the only one which for him is logical but at the same time unbearable: ". . . I have decided to cope with this all by myself."

In terms of survival strategy we could say that Eric chooses a way which shrinks his scope of action. The homophobic tension, shown in his reaction pattern, prevents him from accepting help, chiefly because he chooses to interpret other people's motives of giving help from this point of view. On the other hand, the surrounding world–above, all the doctors–were not capable of understanding his problems. The doctors have probably learned–for one thing because of their close and sensitive cooperation with the homosexuals' own organizations–that the support of homosexual people should come from those who are homosexual themselves. The problem in this case, however, is that the individual concerned does not regard himself as homosexual. The effect of that kind of support that Eric is offered is counterproductive. From the position he has earlier had in the margin of the homosexual social world he is driven more and more out into the periphery and is difficult to get hold of even for people who care for him (e.g., his sister and other friends).

"A Fairly Decent Life"

Henrik (44) tells us the following:

I have lived a quiet life, a life differing from the usual image of homosexuals, doing nothing but having sex with each other. My life is quite the contrary of this, really. I haven't had many relations. Four years ago I fell in love with a chap in Gothenburg and moved to that city but we split up soon after I had arrived there. It was a great disappointment.

In fact, there have been one-night stands mostly, periodically. Once in a while I have been to a disco but I never felt at home in that environment. It's noisy, smoky and messy and it's difficult to make contact with people. When I think about it, it's just as if my own sex life has varied over the seasons. It has always been easiest in the summer. Then you can be out-of-doors, on a beach or in a park. In the winter it has been dull. So when I was just dying for something to happen I went to Copenhagen to go to the baths or a disco and then home again. What an artificial way of meeting others! Being gay you had better be sociable and I'm not.

Actually, in many respects my life has been dull, to speak frankly–the loneliness . . . mainly during my early years. For one thing it was a long time before I admitted to myself that I really was keen on guys. I was 17 or 18 when I made my first sexual contact with another man and at that time I was simply seduced. This was in the early sixties and I found that the homosexuals I met were very peculiar, feminine and superficial, drinking a lot. Their habits were simply different from mine. My interests were much more introspective, I read and studied in all seriousness. And I didn't dare to tell anybody, especially not the family. My mother was awfully negative towards anything that was deviant. She never knew, she died in ignorance, if I may say so.

My father died when I was small. I and my brothers and sisters were never very close. I suppose they thought I was too boring and reserved; I was no doubt. I didn't see my relatives at all. At school I had only a few friends, no real friends, actually. So I lived in a very restricted world. And so it has been, in fact right up to when I was HIV-positive. And maybe a few months after I got the answer.

It was a strange experience when they told me. I was shaken, totally confused, shocked. Actually, it seemed so terribly far-off, for my part. But I remember saying to the doctor that it makes not much difference to me, really. I said so. I sort of meant to say that my life had been so boring even before this happened, so it would not make any dramatic difference for the future. That was how I felt just then and some time afterwards.

Everything became more and more boring, actually. Through the press I was constantly reminded of how many people that were taken ill and how many that died. It was like being at death's door all the time. The last remaining dreams were put aside once and for all, particularly that persistent hope of meeting someone and having a permanent relation. My love life was completely finished. It was painful but also nice in a way. I never had much fun.

Terrible months they were. I realize that now when I think back on it. I got no help from the clinic; I was, in fact, completely alone with all this. Who the hell was I to turn to? It was only me and the papers, everything that was written about that horrible disease, all the accusations that I as a homosexual was lumped together with drug addicts and prostitutes, indiscriminately. Slowly but inexorably I realized what it was all about. In the eyes of the world I was nothing but a second-class citizen; I was promiscuous and a big shit. It became clear to me how amazingly ignorant the surrounding world and the responsible persons of the community were of my and other homosexuals' situation. I was getting more and more angry. My anger was righteous and it sort of forced me away from death's door. A kick in the ass, to be quite frank, and I think that saved me and helped me to be able to live a fairly decent life.

Suddenly it was important to try to get on. I called the RFSL;

they were on duty, and suddenly I was invited to join one of those support groups for HIV-positives that this association was to start up shortly. It was an exceptional step to take, but it was necessary, leaving that paralyzing anonymity. A tremendous experience it was, feeling the security that little group provided. We were only four, including the leader, and we talked about everything under the sun. Surely, they described the homosexual life too sympathetically; I understood that they wanted to pep us up. All the same I have to admit that I was feeling quite fine just then. . .after all these years.

Now, afterwards, I understand that the months in the support group were extremely important to me. First of all, I was given knowledge. I had been so blocked up by all the articles in the newspapers that I hadn't been able to sort out the rubbish, to see what was sensible to stick to. Besides, there was this aspect of time. Suddenly I understood that there was no immediate danger; death was not so imminent. I had some time left, maybe many years. Then I suppose the group-leaders gladly wanted to convince me that I could have sex, too, although being "positive" I didn't find that very convincing, not at that time, anyway.

But I was of course realizing more and more how isolated I had been, and deserted. I started to look up my friends. Well, to be quite honest, I don't think I had looked upon them as friends. You know, I had chosen to define myself as an outsider, an undesirable person. By and by, however, I understood that having good friends was to be the most important thing in the long run. It was simply a question of survival.

What surprised me most of all was the fact that I suddenly sat down and wrote an article to the newspaper on my problem, anonymous indeed, but I did it. It was this about being angry. I was so damned furious at the stupidity that was becoming so widespread in the discussion about the HIV-positives in society and, above all, at the fear of homosexuality which seemed to be beyond reason.

The fact that I wrote that article and had it published was probably more important to me than to the reader. I suppose it was not very original, not very good either, but it was mine; it was I who wrote it.

This happened about a year after I was told that I was HIV-positive. It had been a ghastly year, but for me the most important year, perhaps. Even if I still may feel that it's unfair that I of all people should be infected–I who haven't lived a very dissolute life–I have finally understood that what has happened is of course a result of my way of avoiding life. You must agree, however, that it's damned funny that you have to become HIV-positive to understand what life is all about.

In this story two steps in the adaptation process can be clearly distinguished. In the first step the answer from the hospital was given to a man whose life was characterized by loneliness, disappointment and crushed hopes. It was a highly fateful picture Henrik gave of his homosexual life. It seemed as if homosexuality was something that had come upon him, something he could not help. It had never occurred to him that his homosexual actions might have something to do with choices he made. The way in which he tackled the diagnosis seemed to conform to the same pattern. One might say that his tragic fate was sealed by the virus, which, at the same time, released him, paradoxically, from his responsibility in the future. From now on he was excused from fighting for a better life. The only important thing was to accept the restrictions the infection involved and adapt himself to a life "at death's door."

Henrik's conflict regarding his homosexuality is not a question of "where he belongs" in the first place. Rather, it is a matter of how he looks upon himself as a homosexual. Presumably, this is to some extent connected with his generation. Henrik's cohort group is called "old" in our material, which means that he belongs to those homosexuals who grew up and made their first sexual contacts with other men in the 50s and the early 60s; a period when the idea of "coming out" as a homosexual had not been introduced and when it was quite alien to the great majority of homosexuals to question openly whether heterosexuality was something self-evident (Plummer, 1989). He belongs to a generation of homosexuals who made a point of being unnoticed, a generation in which secretiveness and various strategies of concealing their sexual bias are an integral part of their homosexual form of life. The homosexual life is a life in obscurity conditioned by the heterosexual society.

In this perspective it is understandable that Henrik's negative self-image has served as a self-fulfilling prophesy; in other words, his love affairs have been foredoomed to failure from the very beginning. No more has he been eager to break his isolation except for casual, anonymous contacts in parks and lavatories; surroundings which are extremely hateful to him, because they represent the low value he thinks he possesses in the eyes of the world. For that reason he cannot identify himself with other homosexuals, particularly not with the more "promiscuous" ones. He is not "like that," nor does he want to be regarded as one "like that." This is important to him. Therefore, by emphasizing his individual character in relation to other homosexuals he also claims to be regarded as more normal and, accordingly, more acceptable in the eyes of the world.

Paradoxically, it is the discovery of this false assumption that marks the turning-point in Henrik's process of adaptation and initiates the second step. Being subjected to the picture of AIDS by the mass media, he understands that he is just as contemptible as everybody else who is infected. He is a second-class citizen as any other homosexual. And that is not all; in the eyes of the world he is definitely an outcast, like junkies and whores. When he is seized with "righteous anger," he is forced to act.

Henrik understands that he has to break his isolation to be able to survive. His contact with RFSL is the first step out of "the paralyzing anonymity." Even though he has some difficulty in sharing the firm homosexual identification of the support group, the very reception of him there makes him feel very strongly that he is secure and accepted. He makes friends. "By and by, however, I understood that having good friends would be the most important thing in the long run. It was simply a question of survival."

The article in the newspaper might be regarded as a step in the same direction. True, his views are not expressed openly. The article does not bear his signature. On the other hand the act itself is of great importance to him as a symbolic confirmation of the fact that he has taken an important step to a different, more constructive attitude towards his own and other people's homosexuality. Now he no longer wants to "avoid life," he wants to live. "You must agree, however, that it's damned funny that you have to become HIV-positive to understand what life is all about."

The Turning-Point

The turning-point allows him an increased scope of action, not only for confronting HIV but also for living as a homosexual. One might say that HIV "accelerates" the coming-out process (Plummer, 1975; Lee, 1977; Cass, 1979; Coleman, 1982). At the same time it may be important to observe the facticity of the disease, i.e., the restrictions which it involves and, above all, its time perspective. Even after the acute phase of crisis is over and the time perspective is extended again, most of the men in the study realize that the virus, in all likelihood, will shorten their lives. This knowledge increases their demands on the quality of life during the time which remains. To some of them this will mean that they no longer can hide themselves or "tell lies about who they are." They want to "fulfil themselves" which implies that they want to live a life which they themselves feel is right. In the study there are examples of men who undergo dramatic changes during the phase of adaptation. The developmental work which otherwise would have taken a whole life or never even would have started is compressed into a period of only a few months.

CONCLUSION

Of vital importance to both men's ways of getting along and developing in the phase of adaptation is how they relate to their own homosexuality, i.e., where they are in their coming-out process, in contrast to the acute phase in which such factors as the course of the disease and the social construction of the disease play a more important role.

A more general conclusion that could be drawn from the study as a whole is that those men who live at the center of the homosexual community and practice a relatively "open" homosexual form of life often have at their disposal a social network and other social resources which facilitate an adaptation related to real life. For those who are on the outskirts, living a "covert" life, it is just the other way round.

The men in the study use various strategies in the phase of adaptation for meeting the new demands of a different situation. To some, being HIV-positive is the beginning of a dynamic personal development. This holds true, in particular, of those who decide on a great amount of openness in relation to their homosexuality and their existence as HIV-positive men. This decision is attended by a greater scope of action and thereby greater possibilities of development at all events, as far as I have been able to follow the process through the men's own stories. Particularly remarkable was the fact the HIV-infection accelerated the coming-out process in certain cases. To some of these men, who had had a bitter and ambivalent feeling regarding their homosexuality, the knowledge of being infected with a fatal virus suggested dramatically a "now or never" attitude. The intense and repressed desire for giving full expression to their homosexuality, or at least not having to be ashamed of it, before themselves or other people, were–paradoxically–made possible to satisfy only after they had become infected.

There are, however, also examples of men who come to what rather might be characterized as a deadlock in their development. Their reaction patterns are characterized by a continuous denial of the reality of the infection. It is difficult for them to get out of the acute phase of crisis and they refuse to accept the thought of living with the disaster that has come upon them. These reactions are closely connected with their aversion to regarding themselves as homosexuals. Paradoxically, these individuals are subjected to a twofold process of exclusion; they are stigmatized as homosexuals in the heterosexual majority community while they at the same time feel alien from a more distinct homosexual subculture, which they perceive wants to force them into reconciling themselves to their "true nature" as homosexuals.

The knowledge of these various adaptation strategies is important as a basis of the organization of the psychosocial backing of the HIV-positives. What is a resource to some people is to others a direct hindrance to receiving help. I am referring to the strong homosexual identification associated with the supporting work within many leading voluntary organizations (e.g., Noah's Ark and RFSL). In the study I have seen how this connection to some people is an incentive to liberation while, on the contrary, it seems to work in the opposite direction to others; that is to say, the strong homosexual identification is perceived primarily as something exclusive and reminding them of the fact that they themselves do not belong to "the chosen ones." The men, in whom the HIV-diagnosis produced a strong homophobic reaction, perceive the homosexual support group as a threat; to accept support poses a definite risk of their being labelled as homosexuals. Consequently they prefer to dispense with it. The most important factor as regards the individual's ability of handling a trying situation is the very experience, the value, of knowing that support is obtainable. These men feel there is none. The practical consequence is that they keep to themselves and shrink their scope of action.

It has to be pointed out that the study does not concern itself with a qualified analysis of the actual support systems available for HIV-positives in Sweden. However, it is obvious to most people who have had any experience of the development in this field, both support workers and HIV-carriers, that the quality of psychosocial support is significantly better today compared to the mid-eighties when our men received their diagnoses. In spite of this positive development, it is important to remind ourselves of the implications of our study, emphasizing the need of a flexible supporting system where the HIV-positives should not have to qualify for support by confessing, on false grounds, to a homosexual identity or form of life.

REFERENCES

Cass, V.C. (1979) Homosexual identity formation: A theoretical model. *Journal of Homosexuality*, 4, 219-235.
Coleman, E. (1982) Developmental stages of the coming-out process. *Journal of Homosexuality*, 7, 31-34.
Cullberg, J. (1984) *Dynamic psychiatry*. Stockholm: Natur och Kultur.
Lee, J.D. (1977) Going public: A study in the sociology of homosexual liberation. *Journal of Homosexuality*, 3, 49-78.
Lehne, G.K. (1989) Homophobia among men, in Wimmel and Messner (ed) *Men's lives* (New York, Macmillan), pp. 416-428

Månsson, S-A., Hilte, M. (1990) *Between hope and Despair–a study of HIV and Homosexuality* Lund: Studentlitteratur.

Nilsson Schönnesson, L. (1991) *Stress, adaptation and psychological well-being among homosexual HIV-carriers* Stockholm: Psykhälsan.

Plummer, K. (1975) *Sexual stigma: An interactionist account* London: Routledge & Kegan Paul.

Plummer, K. (1989) Young homosexuals in England, *Lambda Nordica*, 1, 4-39.